WHERE HAVE ALL THE
Nurses Gone?

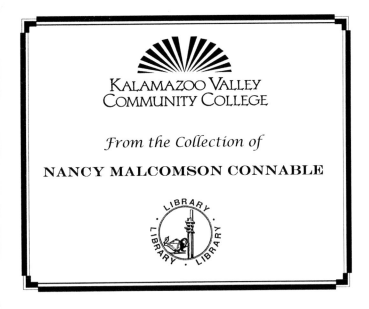

FAYE SATTERLY, R.N.

WHERE HAVE ALL THE

Nurses Gone?

THE IMPACT OF
THE NURSING SHORTAGE
ON AMERICAN HEALTHCARE

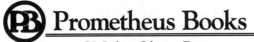 **Prometheus Books**

59 John Glenn Drive
Amherst, New York 14228-2197

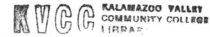

Published 2004 by Prometheus Books

Where Have All the Nurses Gone? The Impact of the Nursing Shortage on American Healthcare. Copyright © 2004 by Faye Satterly. All rights reserved. No part of this publication may be reproduced, stored in a retrieval system, or transmitted in any form or by any means, digital, electronic, mechanical, photocopying, recording, or otherwise, or conveyed via the Internet or a Web site without prior written permission of the publisher, except in the case of brief quotations embodied in critical articles and reviews.

Inquiries should be addressed to
Prometheus Books
59 John Glenn Drive, Amherst, New York 14228–2197
VOICE: 716–691–0133, ext. 207
FAX: 716–564–2711
WWW.PROMETHEUSBOOKS.COM

08 07 06 05   5 4 3 2

Library of Congress Cataloging-in-Publication Data

Satterly, Faye.
  Where have all the nurses gone? : the impact of the nursing shortage on American healthcare / Faye Satterly.
       p. cm.
  Contents: A nurse's life—Where have all the nurses gone?—One day in the life of a hospital executive—Hospital economics: how nurses were lost—Nurses & doctors—And what about the patient?—Enhancing the workplace: how hospitals retain nurses—Nurses: creating solutions—Accountability for health: it's not just for healthcare providers—Advance directives: communicating your wishes—Liability and healthcare—Three West revisited.
  Includes bibliographical references and index.
  ISBN 1–59102–140–5 (alk. paper)
  1. Nurses—Supply and demand—United States. 2. Nursing—United States.
I. Title
  [DNLM: 1. Nursing—manpower—United States. 2. Nursing—trends—United States. 3. Nurse's Role—psychology—United States. 4. Nursing Staff, Hospital—United States. 5. Physician-Nurse Relations—United States. WY 16 S253w2003]

RT86.73.S288 2003
331.12'91362173'0973—dc22

2003021539

Printed in the United States of America on acid-free paper

Contents

Acknowledgments

I t is impossible to write a book about nursing without the support and input of others in this profession. I owe a special debt of gratitude to the nurses, doctors, staff, and especially the patients of Martha Jefferson Hospital, who helped me appreciate how such a difficult job can bring so much joy.

To Nancy Maloy, Janet Silvester, Rob Pritchard, Amy Black, Dorothy Somerville, Kathleen Phalen Tomaselli, Ann Nickels, Becky Owen, Janice Lugar, Carol Vincel, Sylvia Hendrix, Cindy Spaulding, Susan Cabell Mains, Greg Cline, Alice Staples, Mary Scher Baxter, Sam Morgan, Susan Rives, Rob Graham, Dana Trom, Tom Cogill, Joan Maher, and Suzanne Smith, thanks for your friendship, teasing, listening, suggestions, and inspiration. A special thanks to Andrea Wistar, personal coach (and friend), for helping me stay on task.

I am very grateful to Kathleen Valenzi (High Priestess), David Ronka, Ross Howell, Ginger Moran, Charlie Gleason, Lynn Woodson, Matt Genson, and Roussie Jacksina of the writer's group, for sharing their writing expertise.

A special debt is owed to Barbara Blakeney of the ANA; Linda H. Aiken, Julie Sochalski, and Nancy Khan of the University of Pennsylvania's Health Outcomes and Policy Research Center; Jeanne Sorrell of George Mason University; Fran Bonardi and Matt Lambert (all of whose well-earned titles appear in the text) for generously sharing their time and/or their expertise.

And finally, a very special thanks to my favorite, only daughter Caroline Sullivan for listening, reading, editing, and cheerleading; to Frank Gaddy; and my parents, Bill and Vivian Satterly, my sister, Karen Staples, my brother, Don Satterly, and their families for putting up with me.

Writing is only a small part of producing a book. The assistance of the Infusion Nurses Society, especially Debbie Benvenuto, was invaluable. Thanks to my agent, Kristen Auclair, for her representation and advice; to Steven L. Mitchell, editor in chief, for his many thoughtful suggestions; and to the fine team at Prometheus Books for their incredible attention to detail.

Introduction

Nearly two years before writing this book, I sat down to lunch in the hospital cafeteria with a nurse I had known for years. She has long been my ideal of what a good nurse should be. Though she possesses many years of experience and has been offered other positions, she remains steadfastly at the bedside. Always looking for new challenges, she is respected for her clinical expertise and is well liked by other staff, the doctors, and patients. We chatted about hospital gossip until the conversation eventually drifted to our children.

"Your kids must be about college age," I said. "Are any of them going into nursing?"

She laughed. "I told my oldest that I would pay for her entire college education if she chose anything *but* nursing."

Coming from her, the answer was especially surprising. Surely a nurse as dedicated as she would want her children to follow in her footsteps. Then she asked about my daughter and I had to acknowledge that I hadn't nudged her toward nursing either. If anything, I had discouraged the idea. And yet, I loved nursing, didn't I?

The conversation haunted me in the months that followed as rumors of a nursing shortage grew. Alarming statistics were reported in nursing journals and echoed in the headlines of major newspapers. I learned that there were 126,000 vacancies for hospital nurses nationwide, the equivalent of a small city. The national nursing vacancy rate for hospitals and nursing homes had risen to 13 percent. Though some states, such as California, Arizona, Texas, Nevada, and Florida, were harder hit than others, there were few areas that did not feel the pinch. Large medical centers and community hospitals in cities and rural areas all noted that nurses were becoming harder to find. Worse, the average age of the working nurse was forty-five; and since few nurses remain in hospital nursing after their fifties due to the physical nature of the work, retirement was looming. Nursing shortages had happened before, but not like this. Young women, who had historically made up the bulk of the nursing profession, faced unlimited career opportunities and were choosing to enter other fields. Apparently, my friend and I were not the only ones directing our children away from nursing. A survey of nurses by the American Nurses Association revealed that more than half did not recommend nursing as a career to their friends.[1] And the baby boomers were sliding into their retirement years, a time when their need for healthcare was likely to soar. A study reported in the *Journal of the American Medical Association* projected that by the year 2020, 400,000 more nurses would be needed than would be available.[2] Between 1995 and 2001, the National Council of State Boards of Nursing reported a 29 percent decline in the number of graduates sitting for their national licensure exam.[3]

The impact of a nursing shortage on healthcare was once difficult to measure, but new studies indicate that the nurse's role is vital to a patient's health and safety; when nurses have to care for too many patients, a patient's risk of death following surgical procedures rises by 7 percent per patient. In other words, the patients assigned to a nurse who cares for seven patients rather than four have a 21 percent higher risk of death.[4] Those statistics lend real urgency to the growing shortage. Already in some locales, there were reports of hospitals canceling surgeries or diverting patients to other hospitals because there were not enough nurses to give care.

Hospital and nursing associations sent out the alarm. Congress stepped in with a bill supporting the recruitment of new nurses to the field. Johnson & Johnson committed twenty million dollars to a promotional campaign. Concerned about a shortage, people began asking nurses about their job conditions. The news was disturbing. Many nurses were expressing anger about caring for too many patients with too few resources. In newspapers and magazines, nurses were quoted as saying that the patient acuity (level of care needed) had gone up and that the patients were sicker. I started investigating. Somehow in the few short years since I had transferred into the outpatient area of nursing, everything had changed.

Sicker Patients and Shorter Hospital Stays

Hospital stays had shortened. When patients are admitted to a hospital, nurses create individualized care plans to attend to the whole patient—considering their social, emotional, and learning needs along with their medications and specific treatments. They teach patients about their illnesses and the self-care that is required after discharge. They try to devote quality time to their patients. With the new short hospital stays, the patient still needed an effective plan of care, but where previously a nurse might have had five days in which to accomplish it, she now had to jam a week's work into forty-eight hours. And with the shorter lengths of stay, nursing units had become like revolving doors. A nursing unit might start a shift with a census of twenty-three patients and end with the same number, but twelve of the names could be different. Patients were admitted and discharged so rapidly that as one patient was being wheeled out the door, another was taking his place. In one shift's work, while a nurse might be assigned six beds, she could care for nine different patients, each with health and social challenges that she was expected to discover and manage in half the time.

While hospital stays for some conditions and procedures had shortened, for others the admission had been eliminated. Instead of staying in the hospital, patients had procedures in outpatient units and were sent home the same day. At the same time, advances in medicine meant that certain diseases that had once been fatal had instead become chronic. Patients were living longer, but with more complex conditions. The unwitting result was that while many of the patients were sicker, the nurse caring for them no longer had "easy" patients to balance her assignment. Rather than planning care, the nurse was finding barely enough time to react to crises.

MEDICAL ADVANCES AND TECHNOLOGY

Technology meant to help nursing and enhance patient safety was a double-edged sword. Monitors and IV pumps alarmed to notify nurses of problems, but their sheer number and complexity served to distance the nurse from the patient. So much time had to be devoted to the device itself that less time was left for asking patients the important simple questions such as "How do you feel?" Pumps to regulate intravenous fluids and tube feedings; monitors for arterial pressure, oxygen saturation levels, and cardiac arrhythmias; specialized beds for lifting and weighing or to decrease pressure on already compromised skin; pagers and nurse locator badges for finding nurses were all excellent tools, but time was needed to learn to use them. And new medications that offered physicians other options for controlling high blood pressure, heart disease, and diabetes were being introduced at a stunning pace. Before doling out doses, however, it was the responsibility of the nurses to understand a drug's actions and side effects so they could observe for results; a critical issue that required more of what nurses had the least of—time.

DOCUMENTATION AND PAPERWORK

Documentation was another area getting attention. When patient surveys indicated that pain was an inadequately addressed issue, regulatory and accrediting organizations directed their attention to the nurse. It was no longer considered enough to chart that a patient had pain. Nurses were directed to note the location, duration, level, character, and description of pain as well as any distractions attempted that might turn the patient's attention away from the pain. If a medication was given, the level of relief the patient received and the amount of time it took to achieve it had to be documented on the chart.

In the past, elderly patients who got confused in the night and were at risk of falling were restrained for their safety with cotton waist belts and/or cotton wrist restraints. In the new era, both falls and restraints came under scrutiny. Patients had to be screened for risk factors for falls (confusion, frailty, use of pain medication, etc.), then the measures taken had to be charted (spending more time with the patient, reminding him of where he was and how important it was to get help before getting up to use the bathroom, etc.). Ironically, though a nurse could not apply even the simplest restraint without an order from a physician, prevention of falls was considered the nurse's responsibility. If any restraint (after getting a doctor's order) was applied—even raising all four side rails on the patient's bed—the nurse had to observe and chart the patient's response at least hourly. Although the purpose of the intensified documentation was to better attune nurses to patients' pain and risk of falls while in the hospital, the end result was less time to devote to actual care.

GENERAL WORKING CONDITIONS

Compounding the nurses' work woes were the cost-cutting efforts of managed care organizations. In some hospitals, nurses were laid off and those who remained were forced to work overtime to cover off shifts. In other locales, the number of patients to nurses was reported to be as high as ten to one, well beyond the ideal four to five patients that most nurses recommended. In the Northeast, California, and other areas, nurses unionized and strikes were held in protest of the working conditions. And all the while, hospitals found that increasingly desperate measures had to be taken to find enough nurses to care for their patients.

It is not difficult to understand why nurses are unhappy. The major changes that occurred in their work environment in the 1990s—including a big increase in workload—were all instituted without their input. They feel undervalued, unheard, and worry that they cannot provide safe, adequate care for the patients they serve. According to a study published in *Health Affairs* in October 2002, more than 40 percent of hospital nurses reported being dissatisfied with their jobs. One in three nurses under the age of thirty planned to leave their current job within the year.[5]

The shortage is a problem that isn't going away. It has taken more than a decade and a variety of factors to create and will require more than just the efforts of hospital administrators to resolve. It will require assistance from physicians and support from the public, and some of the issues will need to be addressed by the nursing profession itself, particularly the overwhelming reticence of its members to communicate to others the value of their work.

To begin, it is important to sort through the layers that exist within nursing that contribute to the public misperceptions about a nurse's role in healthcare. The term "nurse" applies to a broad group of people and includes a wide variety of positions with varying levels of education and expertise. There are many routes to becoming a nurse and the programs and training are not uniform. Physicians, for example, are all educated in the same way. Each has to attend college, then four years of medical school followed by an internship. It is after that that specialization takes place. One specialty may require a short residency, another may require a lengthy one, but they all begin with the same basics.

TRAINING FOR NURSING

In nursing, however, training is variable. Licensed practical nurses (LPNs) or licensed vocational nurses (LVNs) as they are called in California and Texas, are trained in twelve-month programs at technical/vocational schools, community colleges, or hospitals. They usually provide basic bedside care under the direction of physicians or registered nurses (RNs). RNs may be trained at two- or three-year hospital-based diploma schools or at two- to three-year community college–based associate's degree programs. In both instances, the students are trained to provide direct care, such as administering medications, under physician direction. At four-year bachelor of science programs, RNs are trained to provide direct care, but are also prepared for entry into master's degree (MSN) programs. At a master's level, RNs are trained in leadership roles or to be educators or researchers. Clinical nurse specialists (CNSs) who serve as educators on nursing units and nurse practitioners (NPs) who often work in physicians' offices and have been granted prescriptive powers by some states are trained in master's degree programs.

SPECIALIZATION AND CERTIFICATIONS

Even within the same basic category of training there may be important differences and specializations. The clinical ladder is a means of promoting hospital nurses without removing them from the bedside into an administrative position. Levels are designated by number. A Clinical I nurse may be an entry-level RN, whereas Clinical IV nurses are considered autonomous in their decision-making abilities, able to direct less experienced nurses in their work, are expected to seek and promote educational opportunities, and usually hold at least one certification from a national nursing specialty organization.

Because of the complexity of patient care, specialization within nursing has become important, fostered by specialty nursing organizations. The Infusion Nurses Society, for instance, is a specialty nursing organization that offers not only educational opportunities for nurses to learn about the unique practice of administering intravenous infusions, but a certification exam testing that knowledge. The exam covers infection control practices of infusion therapy, knowledge of chemotherapy for cancer, devices and equipment used for intravenous therapy, infusions for pediatrics (children), as well as blood and blood-product transfusions. Nurses are not allowed to take the exam until they meet a minimum number of hours of experience in the specialty. A nurse who successfully passes the exam earns the initials CRNI (certified registered nurse in infusions) as part of her title to indicate her expertise. There are certifications for operating room nurses, critical care nurses, emergency room nurses, and oncology nurses, just to name a few.

Specialization is needed in nursing in this technological age, but it, along with the variability in training, adds to the complexity of the nursing shortage. A nurse who is fully trained in one area may be unable to function competently in another. This becomes problematic because while a hospital may average a 13 percent vacancy rate in nursing, it is unlikely that it is evenly distributed. The vacancy in the obstetrics (maternity) unit may be only around 5 percent, while the vacancy in the operating room (OR) may hover around 20 percent, but without extensive extra training, the obstetrics nurse can't help in the OR.

EXPERIENCE AND MENTORING

Because of the relatively short time needed to train a nurse, it would appear that the nursing shortage could be quickly solved by enhancement of working conditions and aggressive recruitment of new students into nursing programs. With a significant increase in school enrollment, new graduates can begin filling hospital vacancies within a few short years. The first barrier encountered in that plan is the shortage of qualified nursing instructors, which has limited nursing school enrollment. The problem goes deeper, however. Though training for RNs can be relatively short, it is only the beginning. New nurses need years of experience and mentoring to fully develop their skills. What is apparent to the public is often only the kindness and caring associated with nurses. What is less visible but essential to patients' well-being is the sophisticated level of knowledge and experience utilized in their care that helps prevent complications or allows for quick intervention if a complication occurs. With the aging workforce, it is projected that within a few short years, retiring nurses will be leaving at a faster rate than they can be replaced, leaving behind not just too few nurses, but too few nurses with too little experience.

DEMOGRAPHY OF NURSES

A snapshot of the profession is taken every four years by the National Sample Survey of Registered Nurses, providing important insight into who makes up the nursing workforce. As of 2000, there were nearly 2.7 million licensed RNs. Around 95 percent were women, 87 percent were white, and 72 percent were married. Their average age was forty-five.

About equal numbers—34 percent each—had a bachelor's or associate's degree; 22 percent were diploma school graduates; and 10 percent held a master's or doctoral degree. Nine percent were thirty years of age or younger, compared to 1980 when 25 percent were under thirty.[6] It becomes immediately apparent that opportunities exist in the recruitment to the nursing profession of men, diverse populations, and of younger people.

THE ROLE OF THE PUBLIC

It is important to note that while the nurses' plight can be traced to decisions made by hospital administrators, actions or inactions of physicians, mandates by hospital oversight groups, and to the nursing profession itself, the public has also played a large role. As new technology and medical advances are introduced, the public demands more from healthcare while accepting less personal responsibility for general health. Many of healthcare's limited resources, such as nurses, are being used to forestall inevitable deaths or to correct preventable health problems. A full 65 percent of Americans are overweight or obese, millions still smoke despite the known risks, and an even larger group participates in no regular program of exercise. Less than a quarter of the population utilize their right to create advance directives that outline their wishes for end-of-life care. The implications are astounding. In 2001, healthcare costs accounted for 14.1 percent of our gross domestic product, more than most other industrialized nations. To reverse the trend, our efforts must go into prevention rather than repair and some of the responsibility should be shifted back where it belongs, on each of us as individuals.

A CALL TO ACTION

Though clearly nurses need help and the public needs to know of their plight, writing a book about it felt risky, for it is possible that while I might shed light on this important issue, potential nurses may be frightened away by news of the current conditions rather than drawn to the profession for its incredible rewards. But the more I listened to nurses, the more vital it seemed that their stories were told. Not that they weren't expressing some terrible feelings of being burned out and worn down, but that they were still expressing the same shining desire to "make a difference." They still loved their profession, even if they were discouraged by the demands of their jobs. And when I told nurses about my desire to write this book, they generously shared their opinions, their stories, and their ideas. The Infusion Nurses Society kindly allowed me to distribute my survey at its May 2002 annual meeting. More than 170 nurses returned the form and, with their commentary, added greater insight into the conditions under which they were working. When I called the American Nurses Association, the president, Barbara Blakeney, RN, agreed to be interviewed. And I learned that nurses were taking action. Nurse-friendly magnet hospitals were sprouting up all over the country, while groups like the ANA were lobbying Congress for passage of the Nurse Reinvestment Act and nurse researchers were quantifying the value of nursing in ways that even accountants could understand.

Nurses and the important work they do everyday are inspiring. Whether it is in creating clinics for the homeless, helping patients to die with dignity, learning new ways to take care of stroke and heart disease patients, or teaching patients about caring for their health, the care provided by nurses is vital to the health of the nation. It is difficult to imagine a hospital, clinic, nursing home, or physician's office without a nurse to facilitate the patient's care and safety. But the ailing profession needs attention to survive the current crisis. Within some enlightened workplaces, nurses are already redefining their practice and redesigning their workplaces for optimal care. But more will need to be done to entice young people into the nursing ranks. The real value of their work will need to be recognized and rewarded, a task that is best not left just to politicians and corporations, but to those who will benefit the most—all of us who may one day need care.

Chapter 1 invites you to experience a day as a hospital nurse.

Notes

1. "The ANA Staffing Survey," American Nurses Association [online], nursingworld.org/staffing [February 2002].

2. "Nursing Shortage Fact Sheet," American Association of Colleges of Nursing [online], www.aacn.nche.edu/Media [January 15, 2003].

3. Ibid.

4. Linda H. Aiken et al., "Hospital Nurse Staffing and Patient Mortality, Nurse Burnout and Job Satisfaction," *Journal of the American Medical Association* 288, no. 16 (October 2002): 1991.

5. "Nursing Shortage Fact Sheet," American Association of Colleges of Nursing.

6. Robert Steinbrook, "Nursing in the Crossfire," *New England Journal of Medicine* 346, no. 22, (May 30, 2002): 1761.

CHAPTER ONE

A Nurse's Life

Karen Hensley* stepped off the elevator into the darkened halls of Three West and breathed in the familiar hospital smells. It was 6:30. She was early, but it was her first day as the shift charge nurse, the coordinator of the nursing and support staff who would give care on her unit that day. She was responsible for ensuring that physician orders were communicated and carried out and for assigning the nurses and the nurses' aides to their patients. She wanted time to review the room assignments before the rest of the staff arrived. She liked Saturdays. They were more relaxed than weekdays; patients had fewer tests and procedures, the operating room was open only to emergencies, and the doctors had time for questions since they didn't have office hours awaiting them. The day had potential. She flipped the light switch and watched the hallway illuminate.

"Hey," called Carol, the night shift charge nurse, "are we ever glad to see you. It's been crazy. The supervisor called and said to tell you that Melinda isn't coming in." She held out the assignment sheet with a line slashed through Melinda's name.

Karen stared at the sheet. "What's the census? Are we still full?"

"There's a bunch of discharges expected this morning, but you'll probably fill the beds as soon as you empty them. Flu season." Carol said.

---

*Karen and all the characters in this chapter are fictional, though the daily challenges they face are real.

21

"Who is the supervisor? Did she say she was sending help? We can't take care of all these patients without another nurse or at least an aide."

Carol shook her head. "You don't get it, do you? They don't care."

Karen didn't bother answering. The phone rang and she reached for it. "Three West, Karen speaking."

It was Alice, the nursing supervisor. "Did Carol tell you about Melinda? Her baby's sick and the other bad news is that one of the unit clerks called in, so I'm afraid you'll have to share Elizabeth with Five West."

Karen looked doubtfully at the desk from which the unit clerk, Elizabeth, efficiently managed the unit. "We were already short a nurse before Melinda. We need Elizabeth to help answer call bells."

"Sorry, it's the best I can do. This is your first day in charge, isn't it? Call me if you need anything."

The connection broke. Rachel, a young registered nurse arriving with coffee cup in hand, looked over Karen's shoulder for her assignment. Karen shook her head. "Don't bother. Melinda's called in, so I'll have to reassign her rooms."

Twenty-nine patients, three empty beds, and four nurses and a nurses' aide on patient care—Karen didn't like the math. Instead of a barely manageable assignment of six patients, they would each have to take seven with one nurse taking eight. Seven of the patients were unable to feed or bathe themselves and required total care. Five were only one day post-op (out of surgery) and would need extra attention and teaching about their surgical wounds and what they could do to prevent post-op complications; three were on isolation precautions requiring that the nurses don gown, mask, and gloves each time they went into the room; and one was beginning the alcohol abuse protocol. He was the wild card. The medications authorized by the protocol could help him sleep through the worst of his withdrawal or he could become frightened and confused, even hostile.

The staff had its own issues. Rachel was a new RN and had just finished her twelve-week orientation to the unit. Both she and the licensed practical nurse, Donna, while eager, would require a lot of direction. Emma, another RN, was a solid, steady performer, but Lilly, who was the most experienced, was also the most unpredictable. Her chronic complaining could negatively impact the whole unit. And then there was Ralph, the aide. He was fast, but he couldn't possibly be in all the places he would be needed at one time. With so many total-care patients, he would be kept very busy.

Karen studied the sheet and tried to decide on the most equitable division of assignments. It was nearly 7:00 A.M. before she entered the conference room where Carol was waiting to give her report on the current status of the patients. The small room was tense. Lilly snapped at Karen as soon as she walked in. "Seven patients to one nurse is just not safe, you know. Not the way they are now. They're a lot sicker than they used to be, a lot more work. They get drugs we've never heard of and don't have time to look up."

Carol was quick to feed her fears. "Yeah, and then there's the man in 310 who's been wandering into patient rooms all night looking for his garage."

"Look, it's going to be a tough day, but we can handle it if we get to work." Karen said. "Lilly, I'll take one of yours so you don't have to have seven and I'll take one other so no one will have to take eight. Here's the assignment sheet. Let's listen to Carol's report and get started." She took a deep breath. The shift was only eight hours long. How bad could it be?

At 7:20 the shift change report ended. Dr. Felton was waiting for Karen. "I ordered a stat hematocrit (a NOW order for a lab test measuring the percent of iron-carrying red cells present in a patient's blood) yesterday on Mr. Helmsley and the results aren't on the chart." He held it out to her accusingly.

"Did you try looking it up in the computer?"

Emma interceded as his face turned scarlet. "Here, Dr. Felton, I'll check for you," she said, and led him by the elbow to an available computer monitor.

Elizabeth was whispering in Karen's ear. "Are you crazy? He hates the computer."

"He doesn't have a choice. It's the system we use."

"Yeah, well, I don't want to be around when you break it to him."

Rachel rushed to the nurses' station. "Quick, is Mr. Turner a DNR [Do Not Resuscitate]? I can't find a pulse."

Karen grabbed his chart from the rack and skimmed the order sheet. "Doesn't say. Elizabeth, tell the operator to announce the code, then call his doctor and find out if we should code him or not. Rachel, grab the cart."

Feet pounded down the hall as "Code 12" was sounded over the loudspeakers. The room filled with members of the Code 12 team even as Karen was checking for breath sounds and a heart rate.

"Who is this? What's his diagnosis? Is he a full code?" asked the emergency room physician who had responded to the code.

"Joseph Turner, admitted yesterday from a nursing home with possible pneumonia. Rachel found him without a pulse when she was making her morning rounds. We don't have a DNR order," Karen explained.

The back board (a hard surface placed under an in-bed patient prior to chest compressions to prevent the patient from sinking into the mattress with every push) was put in place and chest compressions started as the ambu bag squeezed air into his chest. The doctor called orders and a nurse from the Code team responded by administering emergency medications through the patient's IV line.

Jim, the respiratory therapist, spoke up. "What was his status before this? Mentally alert? Ambulatory? Is he going to have any quality of life if we bring him around? We'll have to use our last available ventilator and go on Emergency Divert (turning away emergency heart or respiratory patients to other hospitals) to keep him alive."

"I've never seen him before this morning," Rachel said.

"Me neither," said Karen. "I was off yesterday."

The ER doctor frowned. "Get his physician on the phone."

"I just talked to him," Elizabeth said, as she poked her head into the room. "He said he hadn't discussed resuscitation with the family. He'll call the son and get back to us."

Jim's face reddened. "He should have done that before he admitted him. What is he, in his eighties? If the man had no quality to his life anyway, we should be letting him go in peace."

"Clear!" a nurse called as she discharged an electrical shock to the man's chest through the paddles.

Five minutes passed before Elizabeth returned. Five minutes during which the heart was again shocked, more drugs were pumped in, and a tube was passed down the patient's throat for breathing.

Elizabeth's face reappeared. "The son wants us to do everything we can."

Jim was growling. "Does he know what everything means? It's been ten minutes and his heart still isn't beating on its own. So does he want us to continue pounding the old man's chest?"

"We'll give him a few more minutes," the ER doctor said.

The code continued. The nurse doing chest compressions shook her arms out as another moved in to replace her. More shocks were administered, but the EKG monitor showed no sign of an independent heartbeat.

Elizabeth stuck her head through the doorway. "Mr. Turner's son is here. Can he come in?"

The ER doctor disengaged himself. "I'll come out and talk to him. How many minutes now?" he asked the team member recording the proceedings.

"Twenty-two."

"Continue compressions." The doctor followed Elizabeth into the hallway, pulling the door closed. In a moment he was back. "We'll call it. Time of death is 7:56. Jim, why don't you go ahead and pull the tube? Clean him up as best you can. Mr. Turner's son wants to say good-bye."

Rachel was removing the electrodes from the elderly man's chest as the younger Mr. Turner approached the bedside. He gently took his father's hand and spoke in a quiet voice to no one in particular. "I didn't even know he was sick. The nursing home left a message, but I was out of town. I only got it this morning. Did he suffer?" He choked on the last question and the tears started.

Karen touched his arm. "We think he passed in his sleep. We tried to revive him, but he never came around. Why don't we go get you something to drink and let the team get their equipment out of the room? We've got a quiet place if you need to call someone. Then you can come back and sit with your father if you'd like. We're very sorry for your loss, Mr. Turner."

Charts with new orders were starting to stack up on the desk as the doctors made morning rounds. "Who's in charge here?" a surgeon growled.

"I am," said Karen, returning to the desk.

"I ordered a dressing change on Mrs. Garrett last night. It's saturated and making a mess of her bed. Get it taken care of and then I want you to find the nurse who should have changed it last night and write her up." The chart slammed down on the desk and he was gone.

"Karen, I need someone to check this blood with me," called Donna.

Lilly was scowling. "Karen, the pharmacy sent up the wrong drug for Mr. Getshell in 306. And they're saying I need to fill out some form to get it corrected. I don't have time to fill out a form. He wants his medication now."

"Tell him you have to follow procedure, that we do it to ensure his safety, and you'll bring it as soon as you can." Karen said firmly. She started down the hall after Donna, but Elizabeth was calling her name. "Karen, Mr. Johnson's family is on the phone. They want to know how he did last night. . . . Hey!" Elizabeth dropped the phone and grabbed at the arms of the patient on the alcohol abuse protocol. He was seated in a geriatric chair with an attached tray (much like a baby's high chair) and had slid down in the chair. His chin was on the tray, his arms flailed above his head and his bottom hung off the edge of the seat as his private parts escaped the confines of hospital gown to dangle in the fresh air. "Hey, I need a little help here."

A nearby physician rushed to their aid as Karen and Elizabeth loosened the tray and tried to right the patient. "Are you okay, Mr. Templeton?" Karen asked the patient in the chair. "Where were you trying to go? Did you need to go to the bathroom?"

Mr. Templeton rubbed his hand over his face. "The garage, just wanted to go to the garage."

"Do you know where you are, Mr. Templeton? You're in the hospital." Karen patted his shoulder while she spoke over his head to Elizabeth. "We need a waist restraint belt. Can you pull the paperwork for the restraint protocol when you get a chance? After we get him tied down, I'll have to call his doctor for an order."

"It's Mathers. He doesn't like his patients restrained."

Karen was getting exasperated. "Then he can come and baby-sit, 'cause I don't have time."

The phone rang again. It was Mr. Johnson's sister, upset that she had been left waiting on the phone. Karen took it. "Yes, ma'am, I'm sorry that you were left holding. Yes, Mr. Johnson had a good night and is resting comfortably at the moment. Uh huh. Yes, I'll tell him you called."

Another phone line rang. Elizabeth held out the receiver. "Karen, it's Alice for you, but you better hurry, 'cause Templeton is trying to slide down under the tray again."

Together she and Elizabeth got the man seated properly. While Elizabeth went to find a waist restraint, Karen took the call.

"Yes?"

"How's it going?"

Karen didn't reply.

"Did you remember to call the eye bank on Mr. Turner?" asked Alice.

"The eye bank?"

"Yes, we have to call the eye bank on every death. It's in the procedure book. Did his family give you a funeral home yet? If you know which one, I'll call them. Have any idea when you'll get him down to the morgue?"

Karen saw Rachel coming into the nursing station. "Rachel? Did Mr. Turner's son leave yet? The supervisor wants to know when the body will be ready to go to the morgue."

Rachel looked close to tears. "I haven't even seen all my living patients yet. It's nine o'clock. I haven't gotten vital signs and I don't even know if everyone had breakfast. How am I going to have time to fill in all the paperwork for the morgue? And who is going to bring the morgue stretcher and help me lift him?"

"I've got to go," Karen said and hung up the phone. She looked for Elizabeth, who was already headed down the hall, calling out as she walked, "I'll get the stretcher."

"Elizabeth will help. I can help lift when you're ready. Just do the best you can. Maybe we can find an orderly to go with you to the morgue."

A woman, obviously frightened, approached the desk. "My husband is breathing too fast. He says his chest hurts. It's just like when he had his heart attack. He needs the doctor now."

Karen directed the patient's nurse, Emma, into the room for an assessment while she checked his chart for medication that might address chest pain, but there was nothing.

"Emma," she called out, "find out if he's had these episodes at home and if he takes anything for it." She dialed the answering service to alert the physician on call. Emma returned to the desk to report that his vital signs—blood pressure, heart rate, and respiration—were indeed elevated. Five minutes passed and no physician returned the call. Karen called the answering service again. The wife returned to the desk, more frantic this time. "Where is he? He needs to do something now."

"We're waiting for him to call. Emma will give your husband oxygen to make him more comfortable."

Five more minutes passed. Karen's own vital signs were becoming elevated. She paged the nursing supervisor. The wife was getting agitated. "Where is the doctor? He needs the doctor."

The supervisor appeared at the desk. "Is his doctor on call or is somebody else covering for him?"

"He's Dr. Heffner's patient, but Dr. Jennings is covering."

"Never mind. Get the phone book and we'll try Dr. Heffner directly."

Another physician making rounds assessed the situation and interceded with the wife while Karen dialed Dr. Heffner. She braced herself as she heard it ring. She knew he wouldn't be happy. "I'm not on call," were his first words, but he listened to her report, ordered a Stat EKG, nitroglycerin tablets, and promised to be there within ten minutes. Disaster averted.

A new face appeared at the desk, obviously disturbed. "My mother's breakfast is sitting by her bed stone cold. No one's fed her. Or changed her. Her bed is soaked and smells as if there's more there than just urine. What kind of place is this? She can't get to the bathroom by herself, you know. I have never in my life. Don't you people even care?"

Karen stared at her blankly as Elizabeth came to her rescue. "This is Mrs. Bedford's daughter, in 304? I think she's assigned to you today."

"Oh no, I'm so sorry. You're right, we've had a couple of crises this morning and your mother did get forgotten. Elizabeth, see if you can get Mrs. Bedford a fresh breakfast tray."

Karen's shoes burned a trail down the hall.

Noon came and went. Karen had three pieces of chocolate from a box left by a patient's family as he was discharged. She didn't ask what anyone else had for lunch because she knew they had no time to eat.

The patient in 312 lost his dentures, starting a frantic search until a family member acknowledged taking them home for safe keeping.

The nursing supervisor visited the desk to tell Karen that someone would need to work a double shift to help cover the evening shift.

Intravenous infusion pumps alarmed. Call bells chimed. Phones rang. Doctors left new orders. Karen tried to explain diagnoses, medications, or tests to anxious family members. She fielded complaints and tried to soothe those in pain.

Just as the evening shift was preparing to go in for report, as Karen was beginning to believe the day might finally be finished, Mr. Paulson's daughter demanded to speak with her. She was familiar with Mr. Paulson. It was his ninth day in the hospital with a diabetic foot ulcer. He had had intravenous antibiotics, whirlpool baths, and been to surgery at least twice for incision and drainage and then a debridement (the cutting away of dead tissue to allow the good tissue better opportunity to heal). The outcome had not been positive and a possible amputation loomed in his future. Karen straightened her drooping shoulders and prepared for one more confrontation.

"Are you the charge nurse?"

Karen nodded and attempted a smile that went unanswered.

"My father is Mr. Paulson in room 315. He's leaving tomorrow, but he'll probably be back. Dr. Holloway thinks he will need to have his toe amputated." She pulled a tin from a plastic bag. "Dad wanted me to give these to the nurses. They're chocolate chip. I made them this morning."

Karen could barely contain her surprise. "Thank you. How nice! I'm sure everyone will appreciate them."

"He wants to make sure that if he has to come back, he can come here again. He says that all the nurses here have been kind to him, even when he wasn't so nice himself. He's in a lot of pain, you know, and he's afraid. Will you tell them? Especially Emma and Karen and Lilly, he said. Karen, that's you, isn't it? It meant a lot to him and to me 'cause I couldn't be here as much as I wanted to, with a job and my own family to look after."

Karen mouthed all the right words and walked back to the conference room. She laid the cookies calmly down on the table, looked up at the next shift of nurses awaiting report and burst into tears.

The evening charge nurse reached for a cookie. "Just another day in paradise?"

Karen's story isn't an unusual one. It is replayed day after day in hospitals all across America. The details vary, the players change, but the urgency, the overwhelming workload, and the sense of helplessness are often the same. According to a survey of forty-three thousand nurses in seven hundred hospitals reported in *Nursing Management*, 80 percent feel there has been an increase in the number of patients they are required to treat and 40 percent feel dissatisfied with their jobs.[1] Sadly, 50 percent also reported being verbally abused by patients and/or their families in the past year.[2] Nurses I interviewed added that they often missed meals because they were too busy to take a break. They felt overburdened with paperwork and wondered if anyone in management understood or cared.

Not surprisingly, a nursing shortage is upon us. While every profession seems to wax and wane in numbers, the fluctuation of nurses could have more dire consequences than most. The average nurse is in her midforties and anticipating retirement. At the same time, nursing schools report decreased applicants and fewer graduates. In Arizona, a sunshine state attracting many retirees, the RN vacancy rate was estimated at 17 percent in 2000.[3] Labor shortages of such proportion in any other industry would force a certain slowdown in production and services and a major dent in the bottom line of any corporation. But for healthcare, the implications are even more severe, because its "product" is saved lives.

Ironically, just as nurses are becoming scarce, the need for them is increasing dramatically. Over the next decade, aging baby boomers will swell the ranks of the over-fifty-five population, a group that experiences higher healthcare needs than those in their thirties and forties. Seventy-seven percent of cancers, for example, are diagnosed after age fifty-five.[4] At the same time, rapid advances in medicine have increased longevity. People who reach the age of fifty without any major illness have a life expectancy of over eighty, but longer life comes at a cost. It does not imply a life without illness, just better treatments. And to deliver those treatments, we need more skilled nurses.

In reconsidering Karen's day, it is tempting to start pointing fingers and assigning blame, but it would only serve to mask the real issues. In the current crisis facing the nursing profession, there is no clear villain, any more than there exists any unblemished hero(ine). All of the players in modern healthcare—administrators, doctors, patients, insurers, even the nurses themselves—have contributed to the problem. Conversely, as a group, they also have the power to create the solution.

In the chapters that follow we will consider healthcare from varying perspectives to discover the true and sometimes surprising factors contributing to the declining number of nurses. We'll also consider what we as individuals and as a society can do to ensure that the warm human touch of a nurse does not become a memory.

NOTES

1. "Real RN Feedback," *Nursing Management* (September 2001): 64.

2. Ibid.

3. Larry Cooper, "The Nursing Shortage from Bad to Worse," *Hematology Oncology: News & Issues* 1, no. 9 (October 2002): 19.

4. *Cancer Facts and Figures 2002* (New York: American Cancer Society), p. 1.

CHAPTER TWO

Where Have All the Nurses Gone?

I f Karen were asked about her bad day, she might say that she was worried about whether orders and medications were overlooked and that she had too little time for adequate patient instruction and for mentoring the new nurses. She might admit to awakening in the middle of the night frozen with fear as she tried to remember if she had communicated an important detail to the next shift or hung a new IV bag as she had intended. She might sigh and acknowledge that with no time for meal breaks, the sometimes unexpected death of patients, family members angered over the perceived neglect of their loved ones, piles of paperwork, and an uneasy relationship with many of the physicians writing orders, she sometimes seriously considered changing careers. According to the Department of Labor, there are 126,000 nursing vacancies in hospitals and long-term-care facilities around the country.[1] The stresses illustrated by Karen's day could certainly be to blame.

CHANGING SOCIAL FACTORS

The good news is that for well over a million and a half nurses in this country, the sometimes tough realities of nursing are not enough to drive them away. The pressures are intense and the job dissatisfaction is currently very high for many hospital nurses (as will be explored a little later in this chapter), but the nursing shortage is not simply a result of working conditions. A varied set of social factors external to nursing has led to the scarcity of nurses. The growing population, expanding opportunities, and shifting demographics have all contributed to the rising nurse vacancy rate of 13 percent.[2] Social changes over the latter decades of the twentieth century opened many career avenues to women that were previously reserved for men. With 95 percent of the nursing profession made up of women,[3] it is only reasonable to expect that nursing would be impacted.

Dorothy Somerville, RN, a graduate of a diploma school (a three-year, hospital-based training program) who is now in her mid-fifties, explains it this way, "When I was thinking about a career, I had three choices—teacher, secretary, or nurse. Well, I guess there was a fourth choice," she laughs, "but my mama would have disowned me. I didn't care much for typing and even though I liked kids, I couldn't see myself facing a whole classroom full of them day after day, so nursing was the obvious choice. But it's different for my daughters. They have choices I never even thought of."

Of the nurses interviewed who were born before 1950, most named the same three career options cited by Ms. Somerville. Although they reported happily choosing nursing, it was from a small field of possibilities. But women born after 1970 found themselves in a changed landscape. By the time they came of age, careers had few gender limits. Women who graduated from high school in the 1980s and 1990s and were interested in health and medicine understood that they had options. They could apply to nursing school, or if they preferred diagnostics to the administration of care, they were as eligible for medical school admission as their brothers were.

According to American Medical Association statistics, of the students enrolled in medical school for the 1969–70 school year, a mere 9 percent were women. Compare that to the 2001–02 school year, when women comprised 45.7 percent of the medical school enrollees.[4] The American Bar Association reports a similar trend. In 1971, women comprised less than 10 percent of first-year enrollees in law school. By 2002 that number had risen to 48 percent.[5] A quick survey of the 2001

Department of Labor statistics shows that except for jobs involving very physical labor women have entered nearly every occupation listed.[6]

NEW OPPORTUNITIES WITHIN NURSING

Interestingly, at the very same time that social changes were transforming employment options for women, a whole revolution of change was creating exciting new opportunities within the field of nursing. Whereas thirty years ago, nurses were thought of as generalists, able to serve on any nursing unit, nurses today can choose from a whole menu of interesting options. RNs can specialize in the care of women and newborns, in cardiac disease, medical-surgical nursing, postanesthesia recovery nursing, spinal cord injuries, pediatrics, cancer nursing, organ transplants, operating room nursing, emergency nursing, bone marrow transplants, nephrology (care of patients with kidney disease), infusion nursing (care of patients with intravenous infusions), geriatrics, and critical care, to name a few. And nurses aren't confined to hospitals. There are jobs for nurses in home health, schools, public health, long-term-care and rehabilitation facilities, industry, and even in law firms. As more money is poured into the development of new drugs and therapies, nurses are needed in research to give study medications, assess patients for reactions and results, and oversee the accurate collection of data. The Joint Commission on Accreditation of Healthcare Organizations (JCAHO) employs nurses as surveyors to travel to various hospitals and evaluate levels of care. Pharmaceutical companies employ nurses not only to call upon physicians to detail their products, but also as educators for other nurses in the use of new therapies. Each manufacturer of hospital medical equipment hires nurses to assist with staff education for implementation of their products. Another emerging field is nurse informatics, the application of computer science to nursing science. For any healthcare institution to maintain the incredible volume of documentation and medical records necessary for the JCAHO, Medicare, and other insurers, highly specialized computer software is needed. The implementation of such software often takes years due to each institution's specifications and the complexity of the tasks the software is required to fulfill. Who is called upon to interpret the intricacies of the hospital systems for the programmers of the software? Nurses, of course.

Sandi, of Connecticut, who is a nurse with more than thirty years of experience, works as an independent contractor. With the knowledge she acquired as a nurse, she has been able to develop her own one-person business and turn her expertise into a lucrative and satisfying career. She specializes in infusion nursing and travels regionally to give demonstrations of new products and offer support to other nurses as they learn to use them. The nursing profession, she says, has allowed her the freedom to "make a difference, to help provide consistent, quality care, but on my terms."

Irene from Virginia followed a different path. After spending years in hospital nursing, she was able to transform her experience into a position in a law firm as a certified legal nurse consultant, where she utilizes her strong assessment and analytical skills to consult on medical malpractice cases that involve nursing. She sifts through piles of medical records and depositions, uncovering the facts most pertinent to each case. The lawyer she works with considers her an integral part of his team, indicating that while he knows the law, her nursing experience lets her understand the significance of every small detail of a medical record.

One glance at the classified section of *Advance for Nurses,* a general-interest magazine for all nurses, illustrates the broad employment opportunities currently available to nurses. From birthing centers to psychiatric centers, from public health to infection control, from staff nurse to directors and vice presidents of nursing, from case reviewers for law firms to nurse recruiters for large hospitals, the variety of positions is unlimited, as are the enticements. Listed in the advertisements are such benefits as sign-on bonuses, free parking, on-site daycare, clinical ladder programs (systems of promotion intended for nurses who directly care for patients), and tuition reimbursement. Nurses currently in traditional hospital practice find that they are suddenly valuable commodities elsewhere.

CHANGING DEMOGRAPHICS

Even as the nursing profession diversifies, the large numbers of baby boomers and their parents ensure that the need for competent nursing care will increase. In the U.S. Department of Labor's publication "Occupations with the Largest Growth, 2000–2010," registered nurse is listed third in order of demand. The projected growth is 26 percent, or 561,000 positions between 2000 and 2010.[7] Indeed in the difficult job market of the summer and fall of 2002, the healthcare sector was often listed as one of the few growth areas.

THE JOY OF NURSING

The implication of the impending demographic shift of the baby boomers into old age is great. The shortage of nurses needed to address this aging population is not merely a temporary problem that some quick fix will reverse, but is one that will continue to grow to critical proportions in the coming decade if efforts to recruit new nurses are not started and accomplished immediately. That said, it is also important to note that despite the well-publicized pressure cooker work environment, dissatisfaction is not universally expressed among nurses, or at least not at such levels that the majority of nurses are abandoning their chosen profession. In a survey conducted at the Infusion Nurses Society meeting in May 2002, nurses were asked if they would still choose nursing if they had the opportunity to make a new career choice. Of the 225 nurses surveyed, 178 of them responded, from thirty-seven states and Canada. Despite listing numerous complaints such as too little time, too much paperwork, and too little respect, one nurse summed up the prevailing sentiment in her response. She said that given a second chance, she would choose nursing again, if reluctantly, because there "were still those moments" that made it impossible to give up.

Altruism is a strong motivator for nurses. Despite the aggravation, the skipped meals, and the seemingly endless trail of paperwork, nurses continue to get up and go to work because the satisfaction of helping others often outweighs the frustrations. Hospitals and long-term care facilities require nursing care twenty-four hours a day, seven days a week, regardless of holidays, weekends, or special family events that may be happening. Being a hospital nurse also means becoming more intimately familiar than any lover with the peculiar odors, orifices, body parts, and secretions of another human being. Yet, happily, the work has an addictive draw. Whether as grand as saving another's life, as subtle as observing a smile where there was none or hearing the quieted breath of someone who was writhing in pain, nurses report gaining tremendous satisfaction in helping others back to health or toward greater comfort. It is this kind of intangible reward that keeps nurses devoted to their profession.

On the surveys dispensed at the meeting of infusion nurses, most of the questions were open-ended and nurses were encouraged to write as much as they wished. Many obliged. Without prompting, when asked the greatest source of their satisfaction as a nurse, 81 percent responded "making a difference" or "helping." Another 15 percent defined their helping as "teaching." Of the 73 percent who indicated they would choose nursing again, the reasons cited included a simple "Because I love it," "It's a calling," and "I can't imagine anything else I'd rather do."

For others the questions seemed to inspire a more poetic response. "Nursing is the most dynamic profession I have ever encountered," wrote Susan from Illinois. "It taps into my whole person and challenges me intellectually, emotionally, spiritually, and physically."

Cora wrote, "I've done hands-on patient care, I've taught, and I've mentored. I've seen lightbulbs go on in someone's eyes when they learn something new, I've seen smiles amidst grief and loss and sighs of comfort because of something I did. What other profession could have given me all this?"

Lisa from Arizona was enthusiastic about the variety available in nursing. "There is no other field in which someone can do so many things. I have been with my employer for seventeen years and have done at least twelve different jobs!"

Camille, a nurse for twenty-six years, spoke volumes. "In spite of the drawbacks—intense pressure, constant need for higher levels of learning associated with increased responsibility, sicker patients, lawsuits, less help, and less time—there is still no other profession as rewarding as being a nurse! Where else can you save a life; comfort a mourning spouse, parent, or child; interpret a complicated regimen to a newly diagnosed cancer patient; hold the hand of a dying patient; provide knowledge to the fearful; pray with the shut-in; relieve the pain of a stoic; and act as a patient advocate in a less-than-perfect medical world?"

From the results and comments received in the survey, it appears that despite the current challenges in nursing, the profession itself still inspires unshakeable loyalty. That the Camilles, Susans, Sandis, Coras, and Lisas still exist is the good news for nursing. The sense of altruism that holds them, if valued, nurtured, and publicized, could prove a significant enticement in recruiting for the future.

THE EMOTIONAL COSTS

Sadly, many others responding to the survey indicated that their desire to help has been crushed under what they consider to be unmanageable expectations. And if their disenchantment becomes so great that they retire early or choose another career, there aren't enough fresh young nurses to replace them. In 2000 only 9 percent of registered nurses were under thirty, as compared to 25 percent in 1980.[8] This is particularly bad news for hospitals, because younger nurses are more likely to work in acute-care facilities than are older nurses.

Jane, a nurse with more than twenty years' experience, describes herself as "burned out" on hospital nursing. She shakes her head as she talks and her brown eyes are sad. "I love the patients," she says, "and giving good care, but I don't feel like anyone cares anymore. Do you know how many weekends I've worked over the last twenty years? I didn't really mind, but it seems like with all I've given, I should be getting something back. I mean, all these years. Its seems like I've earned weekends off now so I can still spend some time with my kids before they're gone. So I asked for a few extra weekends and they practically laughed at me. They said that everyone has to work weekends, you know? They can't make exceptions for me. After twenty years, it seems like I should be getting something. Many times I had to work Christmas and Thanksgiving, and I didn't complain. But those people upstairs, they don't care. They don't work any weekends. And you know, the way I feel is making me frustrated with the patients, too. Does that make me a bad person? Maybe it's just time for me to have a change. A regular Monday-to-Friday job like the rest of the world. I wish I'd taken more business courses in school or something."

Jane represents a growing number of nurses who find themselves disillusioned with their career choice. They wonder how much they've given up, if the price they have paid has been worth the reward. Some good, experienced nurses are finding that they are no longer satisfied with their profession. They're looking for a way out of the acute-care setting, and though their words may focus on one area in which they have been mistreated, their feelings are much more diffuse. They are tired, they feel unappreciated and unheard, and they worry about the level of responsibility falling on their shoulders. It is easy to dismiss them as complainers, but it would be more accurate to see them as depressed, "burned out." And it is important that we understand why, because it is their feelings of hopelessness and being overwhelmed that are driving the nursing shortage.

THE EFFECT OF NURSE STAFFING ON PATIENT SAFETY

"Serious Health Risks Posed by Lack of Nurses" read a *Wall Street Journal* headline on May 30, 2002.[9] The headline referred to a study published the same day in the *New England Journal of Medicine* about staffing levels of nurses and their relationship to patient outcomes. The conclusion of the study—the first of its kind—seems obvious: nursing care, specifically the care given by registered nurses, has a positive impact on hospitalized patients. The authors of the study, from the Harvard School of Public Health, Vanderbilt University School of Nursing, and Abt Associates, a policy research and consulting firm, examined data from 799 hospitals in eleven states. They found that a higher proportion of nursing care given by registered nurses (as opposed to LPNs and nurses' aides) and a greater number of hours of care given by registered nurses per day were associated with lower rates of certain types of infections and shorter hospital stays. These conditions were also associated with a 2.5 percent lower rate of "failure to rescue" deaths—deaths that could have been prevented had the warning signs been identified earlier and intervention begun,[10] including pneumonia, shock or cardiac arrest, upper gastrointestinal bleeding, sepsis (an overwhelming and often fatal systemic infection) or deep vein thrombosis (blood clot, usually in the leg).[11]

In October 2002 the *Journal of the American Medical Association* published a study reported by the University of Pennsylvania School of Nursing that corroborated the importance of adequate RN staffing. After reviewing the records of more than two hundred thousand patients who underwent general, orthopedic, or vascular surgery in 1998 and 1999, the researchers concluded that for each patient added to a nurse's workload, the patient's risk of dying within thirty days of admission increased by 7 percent.[12] For example, the risk of death increased to 14 percent if a nurse's assignment increased from four to six patients. The story was covered by all major news outlets, including the evening television broadcasts. To nurses, who were delighted to see evidence that others could comprehend, it was not news. They were already convinced that their work mattered. But the study may offer very important proof to institutions that are considering lowering the ratio of nurses to patients or substituting less-trained healthcare workers for RNs in response to the shortage. It would be wise to put their efforts into more recruiting, for it is apparent that numbers of RNs directly impacts quality of care.

The Joint Commission on Accreditation of Healthcare Organizations, commenting on the significance of the shortage, indicated that nursing "staffing levels have been a factor in 24 percent of the 1,609 sentinel events—unanticipated events that could potentially result in death, injury, or permanent loss of function—that have been reported to the Joint Commission as of March 2002"[13] by healthcare facilities. The report went on to declare that the shortage is "diminishing hospitals' capacity to treat patients" by impacting their ability to see patients in a timely manner in emergency departments and reducing the number of available staffed beds.[14]

It is little wonder, then, that the public is growing concerned. Just prior to announcing its multimillion-dollar nurse recruitment campaign in 2002, Johnson & Johnson commissioned a poll to determine public attitudes about the nursing shortage. The results of the poll indicated that 81 percent of Americans believe that the nursing shortage is a serious health problem; more than half consider it a crisis. They also seem to have a negative view of the nursing work required relative to compensation: while 83 percent indicated that they would encourage a loved one to become a nurse, only 21 percent would consider nursing as a career for themselves. For males who responded to the survey, that number fell to 10 percent.[15]

TWENTY-FOUR/SEVEN

"Do you need a change from clinical nursing? Do you want to work Monday to Friday? Rather than being involved in 'hands-on' patient care, wouldn't you like to see patients from a different perspective?" A flyer with these questions recently appeared in my mailbox alongside the usual bills, credit card offers, and requests for donations. It was a recruitment piece intended to lure unhappy nurses from acute care facilities by aiming at one of their vulnerabilities—a schedule that runs twenty-four hours a day, seven days a week. As discussed earlier, some factors involved in the current nursing shortage are either outside of our control (the aging baby boomers and the population surge of the 1990s) or are actually positive developments (the growing opportunities for women in the workforce). The hours that need covering is yet another factor that cannot be changed. Illness doesn't recognize holidays or weekends and patients' needs do not disappear after dark. That makes it all the more vital to effect changes where possible to ensure that a higher percentage of Americans will consider nursing as a future career and that those currently in the profession will want to remain there. Both are critical issues in raising the number of registered nurses to meet the growing demand.

NATIONAL SURVEYS REVEAL NURSES' PERCEPTIONS OF WORKING CONDITIONS

In a national nursing survey conducted online by the American Nurses Association (ANA) from December 2000 through January 2001, approximately seventy-three hundred nurses offered their opinions about their own working conditions, specifically staffing, patient care, and safety. Most of the respondents worked in a hospital or other acute care facility. More than half indicated that they would not recommend the nursing profession as a career for their children or friends, and 23 percent said they would "actively discourage" someone close to them from entering the profession.[16] Thirty-eight percent reported being "exhausted and discouraged"[17] at the end of a workday, while less than a fifth indicated that they left their shift "exhausted but satisfied."[18] Over a third described leaving work "discouraged and saddened by what they couldn't provide for their patients," and 20 percent actually indicated that they feared for their patients.[19]

Most disheartening is that nearly one-third of the nurses reported feeling powerless to make a change. They remain concerned for their patients, they feel exhausted on a daily basis, but feel hopeless to change things for the better. It is easy to understand the source of Jane's feelings of burnout. The theme of having little control over the environment of care was one that repeated itself in the survey distributed at the Infusion Nurses Society meeting. Several nurses complained of feeling that the care was no longer directed by clinicians, but by insurers, regulatory agencies, and administrators who had business rather than clinical backgrounds. A sense of powerlessness at work is a strong deterrent to new recruits as well, especially with the younger generation. They are looking for not only respect, but balance in their work and home life. Only those with limited choices enter fields where they have little option for self-governance and control over policies such as enforced overtime.

A major source of dissatisfaction for nurses cited in nearly every reference was the increasing time spent on nonnursing tasks, including paperwork and patient transport. In a profession that is not known for its high salaries, flexibility, or optimal schedules, a primary attraction is the opportunity to help others by spending one-on-one time with patients. That makes the next response especially significant: A full 56 percent of the nurses in the ANA survey indicated that the time they had available to spend in direct patient care had decreased while more than 55 percent indicated that the number of patients they were expected to care for had increased. In other words, more work with less time in which to do it. Not surprisingly, three-quarters felt that the care in their institution had declined over the past two years as a result. Though they were feeling increasing pressure to skip meals and work overtime in order to accomplish more, their sacrifice did not seem to have the desired affect. More than 40 percent indicated that they would not feel confident about having someone they loved cared for in the institution in which they worked.

More than two hundred nurses who had left the profession still felt strongly enough about it to respond to the survey. Their top four reasons given for working outside of their field were that their current position was more rewarding professionally, the salaries were higher, the hours better, and while in the healthcare environment, they had feared for their safety.

In another ANA survey posted later that same year on the subject of health and safety in nursing, nearly five thousand nurses responded. Sixty percent reported that they feared a crippling back injury on the job, while 45 percent feared that they would contract hepatitis or HIV from a needlestick injury. A quarter of the nurses feared that they would be assaulted by a patient while at work.

The University of Pennsylvania's School of Nursing's Center for Health Outcomes and Policy Research conducted a much larger study in 1998 and 1999 of more than forty-three thousand nurses in five countries. More than 43 percent of the nurses surveyed scored high on the "burnout inventory," which measures emotional exhaustion and the extent to which a nurse feels overwhelmed by her job duties. Of the nurses surveyed who were less than thirty years of age, one-third indicated that they planned to leave their job within a year.[20]

NURSES' PERCEPTIONS IN THEIR OWN WORDS

The survey given at the Infusion Nurses Society (INS) annual meeting and conference differed from the ANA survey in that it involved a smaller sample—fewer than two hundred nurses—and had open-ended rather than multiple-choice questions. It was also limited to specialty nurses, who often report a more collegial relationship with physicians and greater job satisfaction than generalists. That said, many of the responses echoed those given to the ANA.

Wages Compared to Level of Responsibility

Nearly two-thirds of the INS respondents had been in nursing for more than twenty years, with only 6 percent reporting less than ten years' experience, mirroring national statistics about the declining numbers of young people entering the field. More than half indicated that they earned more than $55,000 annually, with more than a third earning over $65,000. Interestingly, though salary was noted a dozen times as being a source of frustration, it was not about the actual dollars. In fact most of the nurses who mentioned money indicated that they were relatively well paid. Those who said it was not enough felt that it just didn't adequately compensate for the level of responsibility they bore.

When asked if they would choose nursing again, 26 percent of the respondents indicated that they would not. Asked why, one nurse from Arizona wrote simply, "I'm tired." Inadequate staffing was listed as her primary source of frustration (Arizona was reported as the state with the highest estimated vacancy rate in 2000).

Nurses' Desire for Respect

A number of respondents who would not choose nursing again indicated that they still enjoyed healthcare. A handful said that given a second chance, they would choose to be a physician "where I would get more respect and appreciation for what I do." Others wrote that they would consider physical therapy, pharmacy, or radiology rather than nursing, where they felt the "reward is becoming more and more limited."

The lack of respect afforded nurses was listed many times as a source of dissatisfaction. Some pointed the finger at administrators, specifically nonnursing administrators, who directed care without "listening" to the nurses at the bedside or without understanding the complexity of clinical care. Many felt that the "suits and ties" were driven more by the financial bottom line than by the quality of care, a fact that caused them great concern for patient safety. A few mentioned physicians as the main source of disrespect. When asked specifically whether they felt respected by their administrators, only half responded affirmatively. Only a slightly larger number of nurses felt that physicians respected them.

Coming from an institution where relationships between physicians and nurses are mostly positive, I was surprised by the response to the doctor question. However, in a June 2002 article in *U.S. News & World Report*, physician abuse of nurses was reported as a major source of job dissatisfaction for nurses. They reported incidents of doctors' yelling, hanging up on hospital nurses who called to report patient information, and even throwing items.[21] In a survey for the *American Journal of Nursing*, nearly 90 percent of the respondents "had witnessed yelling, public berating of nurses by doctors, and abusive language."[22]

Paperwork

The quantity of paperwork required in recent years was cited in nearly every survey as a means of taking nurses away from their primary responsibility—the patient—with the blame being shared between insurers such as Medicare and regulatory agencies such as the JCAHO. One nurse noted that volumes of documentation were needed to "prove that you're actually doing good nursing."

Holidays and Weekends

Like Jane, the nurses said that schedules requiring long hours and weekend and holiday work were a source of regret. Several nurses indicated that the number of special family events that had been missed and amount of time spent away from their families and children as they were growing up was too great. As one nurse from Florida said, "The many years of working Christmas and all the holidays cost me more personal time with my family than other professions would have."

Personal Safety

A few nurses mentioned that they had fears about both their own potential exposure to HIV, hepatitis, and antibiotic-resistant infections and bringing disease home to their families. A nurse I spoke with who had had a needlestick injury with a "dirty" needle told me of her experience of being tested for HIV and hepatitis B and C and being counseled to have only protected sex with her husband until at least six months after the event to ensure that all tests were negative. She said that was a turning point for her. The incident forced her to rethink the merits of remaining in an acute-care setting; she soon left for an employee health position at a manufacturing plant.

The sheer physical nature of the work was a major deterrent to choosing nursing a second time, said some nurses. They worry that they will be forced to leave their jobs due to injury before they reach retirement age. "It's not just the lifting of patients in bed. It's walking with them down the hall or to the bathroom and suddenly they feel faint. Are you going to let them hit the floor?" And the patients are getting larger. Obesity now affects nearly a quarter of the American public. For nurses who may have to lift or assist patients immobilized by illness or injury, the epidemic of obesity has a significant impact on workplace injuries.

Though no nurses mentioned it specifically in the INS survey, there is another safety issue that is being reported in nursing literature: violence in the workplace. According to a July 2001 article in the *American Journal of Nursing*, nurses have been injured and killed as a result of attacks by patients or criminals seeking drugs and money. Very few hospitals follow strict security measures except on specific units, and often their guards lack the adequate training to deal with someone who really intends harm. According to the author, "working in a healthcare facility is considered to be the third most dangerous job in the United States." At a conference of Emergency department managers in November 2002, more than 90 percent of the respondents pointed to patient violence as the greatest threat to Emergency department personnel.[23]

Liability

A few nurses listed the fear of lawsuits as one reason for not choosing nursing a second time. They said that the additional stress of worrying that suspicious patients were watching their every move was more than they could cope with. One nurse told of the shock of receiving a subpoena with her name on it. Though her lawyer assured her that she was named only because her signature had appeared somewhere in the patient's chart, it did not mitigate her feelings. "The lawsuit came two years after the incident. I had no memory of the patient, his problem, or what he had looked like. I felt totally helpless to even speak in my defense." Though the hospital assumed the liability and the cost of defense, the experience soured her love for nursing.

Not Enough Time with Patients

Though the concerns mentioned so far offer important insights into the current climate in which nurses are working, they are actually secondary issues. Piles of paperwork, understaffing, increased workload, lack of respect, and a sense of powerlessness to effect change are all focused around nurses' primary concern: their growing inability to do what they went into the profession to do—give care. The nurses who indicated that they would not choose nursing again felt overwhelmed with worry by their inability to focus on the patient, to offer the quality of care they knew they were capable of giving and felt their patients deserved. Many of the nurses who had been in the profession for twenty years or more reported that the change had come about only over the last decade.

It is also important to note that of the majority of nurses who would choose nursing again, many echoed the same frustrations as those who would not; implying that they just may not have reached their breaking point yet.

One nurse who left acute care for teaching said it this way, "Sometimes I want to tell my students to run for their lives and do something else. I'm teaching them the ideals of nursing, most of which go out the window shortly after being employed in the real world."

NOTES

1. Robert Steinbrook, "Nursing in the Crossfire," *New England Journal of Medicine* 346, no. 22 (May 30, 2002): 1761.

2. Ibid.

3. Ibid., p.1757.

4. "Table 2—Women Medical School Applicants," American Medical Association [online], www.ama-ssn.org/ama/pub/article/171-196.html [January 2003].

5. "Women at a Glance," American Bar Association [online], www.abanet.org/women/currentglance.pdf [January 2003].

6. "Employed Person by Occupation, Sex & Age," U.S. Department of Labor [online], ftp://ftp.bls.gov/pub/special.req/If/aat9.txt [January 2003].

7. "Occupations with the Largest Job Growth, 2000–2010," U.S. Department of Health and Human Services [online], www.bls.gov/emp/emptab4.htm [January 2003].

8. Steinbrook, "Nursing in the Crossfire," p. 1762.

9. Laura Johannes, "Serious Health Risks Posed by Lack of Nurses," *Wall Street Journal* (May 30, 2002), p. D1.

10. Ibid.

11. Jack Needleman et al., "Nurse-Staffing Levels and Quality of Care in Hospitals," *New England Journal of Medicine* 346, no. 22 (May 30, 2002):1715.

12. Linda H. Aiken et al., "Hospital Nurse Staffing and Patient Mortality, Nurse Burnout and Job Satisfaction," *Journal of the American Medical Association* 288, no. 16 (October 2002): 1991.

13. JCAHO, *Healthcare at the Crossroads: Strategies for Addressing the Evolving Nursing Crisis* (August 2002): 7.

14. Ibid.

15. "Johnson & Johnson Launches Ad, Recruiting Campaign to Reduce Nursing Shortage," Johnson & Johnson [online], www.jnj.com/news/jnj_news/20020418_1558.htm [February 6, 2002].

16. "The ANA Staffing Survey," American Nurses Association [online], http://nursingworld.org/staffing [February 2002].

17. Ibid.

18. Ibid.

19. Ibid.

20. "Study Finds Nurses Dissatisfied," CBSNews [online], www.cbsnews.com/stories/2001/05/07/national.shtml [May 7, 2001].

21. Josh Fischman, "Nursing Wounds," *U.S. News & World Report*, June 17, 2002, p. 54.

22. Alan H. Rosenstein, "Nurse-Physician Relationships: Impact on Nurse Satisfaction and Retention," *American Journal of Nursing* 102, no. 6 (June 2002): 32.

23. "Patient Violence Still Greatest Threat to Emergency Department Personnel," VHA [online], www.vha.com/publicreleases/021121.asp [November 21, 2002].

CHAPTER THREE

One Day in the Life of a Hospital Executive

J erry Standhill* liked to get up early, before the wife, before the kids when they were still home. He would dress in his shirt and tie and suit pants, but leave the jacket folded neatly over the kitchen chair until it was time to leave. Then he would carefully measure the coffee and pour in the water and while it brewed, he would slip out to the deck in the peace and quiet of dawn to watch the sky lighten. He loved that part of the day best. His next favorite moment was when he first stepped into his office at the hospital, his second cup of coffee in his hand. He nearly always arrived before his secretary to enjoy those few moments of solitude when he could dive into the stack of folders on his desk and prepare for the day with a clear head. Some days he started with a 7:15 meeting with one physician group or another, but on the good days, his first meeting wasn't until 8:00.

As he entered his office, jacket over his arm, Jerry thought that there hadn't been a good day in a long time. The phone was already ringing. He had the *Daily Sentinel* folded in his hand, given to him by Shirley, the cafeteria cashier. She was at work by 5:30 every morning, and sometime between the brewing of gallons of coffee and setting up the cereal and muffins, she always found time to skim the headlines. If the hospital had made the paper, Shirley alerted him before the first board member could

---

*Jerry Standhill and the other characters in this chapter are fictional, though the challenges they face are real.

call. Today's headline wasn't one of the good ones. It was about going on emergency diversion; having all the beds in the hospital full and diverting patients and emergency vehicles to the next largest town, fifty miles west. He skimmed the article quickly as he picked up the receiver.

"Jerry Standhill." He said his name as greeting.

"Did you see the paper this morning?" It was Mike Simmons, the president of the board. He didn't bother identifying himself.

"I'm looking at it now. At least he presents facts and doesn't blame the hospital for not having a bigger building." Jerry was frowning.

"Think the television will pick it up? What are you going to say?"

"I'll have Alan in Public Relations work something up. He was working on it last night before we left. He may have e-mailed it to me." Jerry punched on his computer as he talked. "Do you want to take questions if it comes to that?"

"No, I think we should downplay it, don't you? The last time this happened was last year, right?"

They talked for a few more minutes, strategizing about how to handle the publicity and the underlying problem. Just five years earlier, it had looked as if they had too many beds. All the services were moving to the outpatient area, but now the trend was reversing. The population was getting older.

By the time Jerry signed on and checked the messages he'd received since he'd left at 7:00 the night before, his coffee had cooled. He read three letters his secretary, Deborah, had laid on his desk. Two were short thank-you notes from patients about the great care they received. One was a long letter, detailing multiple complaints.

"Mr. Standhill." It was Deborah. He would never be just Jerry to her. "Dr. Beech is on the phone. He's demanding to speak with you. Should I tell him you're in a meeting?"

Dr. Beech was a surgeon. He hated change and held to the belief that the hospital was a "deep pocket" enemy and he was not shy about sharing his opinion. Though it was sometimes a stretch, Jerry tried to maintain a cordial relationship with him. The doctor was the source of many referrals to the hospital and, as such, a major contributor to the revenue stream.

"Do you know what it's about this time?"

"He said something about clamps. I think you got a memo from Joe in Materiels about changing the manufacturer? If I remember right, it was a pretty large cost savings."

"Yeah, but didn't Joe say he had a consensus from the surgeons?"

"He had the support of Dr. Crockett, I think, and Dr. Wise, but I don't remember him mentioning Beech."

"Figures. Give me a minute to put my hand on that memo, and then put the call through." He rifled through a file and located the memo just as his phone rang. "Good morning, Jim," he said by way of answering. He tilted back in his chair and prepared to listen.

"Jerry, this is getting out of hand, when some paper pusher in Materiels can make unilateral decisions about the equipment surgeons use in the OR. And then when I went to find the culprit, he said it was done with your approval. I thought you of all people understood."

"I believe, Jim, that the decision was made with input from several of your colleagues who thought we had found a good substitute. And when Materiels asked you to give it a try so we would have your input, you refused. Now just a couple of months ago, when you wanted to change to the powderless nonlatex gloves, the hospital agreed, but it added about $36,000 a year in cost. So if we can find some ways to make that up, we're going to have to do it, make more economical choices where possible."

"So what did he say to that?" asked Howard, the chief financial officer, while they waited for their weekly operations meeting to start.

Jerry smiled, but it was more reflex than humor. "The usual. Said he knew about all the money the hospital had hidden away, that we were no better than the insurance companies, just trying to get fat off the backs of the workers."

"You'd think that he would have noticed in his own office how much things have changed over the last two decades. There is no fat in the system, at least not on the provider side. I can't imagine he's making more money than he used to."

Jerry shrugged. "No, and that's probably the problem, really. He's scared. The pressure is being ratcheted up on him and he's just trying to control what he can."

The last few stragglers came into the conference room. "Looks like we can start the meeting," Jerry announced, "and we've got a pretty full agenda. Georgia, you have a safety issue you wanted to address."

"Patient restraints." Georgia, the risk manager, said. The whole room groaned collectively. Georgia raised one eyebrow and kept going. "I know you don't want to hear about it; and frankly, I'm tired of talking about it, but JCAHO [Joint Commission for the Accreditation of Healthcare Organizations] doesn't seem to be tired of the topic yet. As you know, a couple of years ago, they beefed up their surveillance on restraints. They said that all hospitals had to have policies that didn't allow nurses to apply restraints without a doctor's orders and that those orders had to be renewed every twenty-four hours. And they dictated how often the nurses had to 'put eyes' on a restrained patient, etc. Well, we did a chart review for the month of November and unless we show improvement, we could be in trouble. That's a Type 1 violation. I'm sure the nurses are doing what they're supposed to, but they've got to document it to prove it."

Said Mary, the vice president for Nursing, "The more time we put into documentation, the less time there is for patient care. We need more nurses."

"Let's not start any talk of adding staff. There's got to be a better way," said Howard, the chief financial officer. "And overtime's up this month, by about 10 percent. That has to be controlled immediately, along with contract help [temporary staffing supplied by an agency at a higher-than-permanent market rate]. I thought we had the hospital staffed so that we didn't need any more contract help."

"I've got the contract help," chimed in Carla, the director of the Lab [department in which tests are conducted on blood and other specimens]. "We've been recruiting everywhere and there are just no medical technicians to be found. The work has to be done, so we had to contract an outside supplier."

"Me, too," added Greg, the Radiology director, "I had two radiology techs go out on short-term disability at the same time. Either we get some contract help in here, or shut down the CT scanner."

"My department is probably responsible for a big chunk of over-time. Remember all that capital expense you put out for us six months ago?" It was Darren from Radiation Oncology. "Well, this month the equipment was finally installed and the staff had to learn how to use it all. We had training for two weeks straight. Half the techs would treat while the others trained and everyone had to work extra to get it done."

"I think we need to get back to Georgia's issue about patient restraints." Jerry interjected. "What are your suggestions, Georgia?"

She laughed. "My specialty is finding the problems. I was hoping this group could find the solutions."

"Seems clear that the nurses just have to follow the guidelines," said Howard.

"They know what they need to do," said Mary, "but no one is telling them how. They already feel like they have less and less time to spend on the things that matter—the patients and their care. They're told not to dare have any overtime without authorization. Half of them are already skipping meals. A break is unheard of. So what would you like them to do?"

"I can't believe that there isn't some area that could be improved upon to give them more time to attend to the things that have to be done." Howard was looking at his report. "Nurses make up the largest group of employees in the hospital. So everything they do has a big impact on the bottom line. With JCAHO issues, the rest of us can all work as hard as we want, but if the nurses don't toe the line, we're done."

"Why don't you come and work alongside one of the nurses for a day? Then you could tell us what changes we could incorporate to increase efficiency," Mary responded.

Jerry interjected. "What about the clinical documentation system we've been talking about? Would that help?"

All eyes turned to Sam, the Information Systems director. He held up his hands. "Don't look at me. I've been advocating for that system for years, but every time I tell you what it will cost, no one wants to hear any more. And you need the whole system so that physicians can enter orders directly and there's no need to decipher their handwriting. Then the medications are barcoded so that nurses can't make mistakes when giving them out, and then there's the clinical documentation part so that all their assessments can be entered as they do them. A physician can come to the unit and instead of searching for a nurse, he can look in the computer and get all the data he needs. Plus, it leaves little room for error. It serves as a constant cue to the nurse about what should be included in her assessment and how it needs to be worded to meet JCAHO standards."

Georgia chimed in. "Pretty soon we won't have any choice. Patients won't want to be admitted to a hospital that doesn't have those systems in place because they so drastically reduce the rate of error."

"But we're talking about a $5-million commitment," said Sam. "And we'll need staff, nurses, and techs who know how we operate who can dedicate their time to building a whole system. It'll take years to complete, and then as we introduce each new piece, staff and physicians will have to be trained to use it."

Jerry shook his head. "This sounds like a discussion for another day. Sam, I think you better call Deborah to organize a meeting with you, Howard, and myself."

"Jerry, since this will impact Nursing most, wouldn't it be a good idea to include them in the preliminary discussions?" Mary asked.

Jerry nodded. "Georgia, it looks like we don't have an answer to your questions, so perhaps you and Mary can get together to discuss?"

Georgia nodded, but when he looked to Mary for assent, she said, "Without more help, there is no answer."

Howard looked dour. "CMS [Centers for Medicare and Medicaid] put out a notice of their April price changes. It was announced as a 4 percent upward adjustment, but once we went over the details, it turns out it means a reduction of about 1.9 percent for us because of our case mix [the percentage of patients who are surgical patients as opposed to suffering from a medical illness. Reimbursements are higher for surgeries than illnesses]. The procedures for which rates were increased we aren't doing, and the ones they're decreasing, of course, we are doing. So we lose." He looked around the table. "I guess I don't have to tell you what that means. We're going to have to find a way to get rid of the contract labor and the overtime. We don't have any choice. We may have to consider a hiring freeze. As people leave, hold off replacing them."

Protests rose from every side of the table.

"Just one of the options we should be considering. We're not meeting the budget. We're only halfway into the year and our costs are well beyond what we budgeted and our number of patient days are down. Length of stay is down."

Jerry listened, but he already knew the tune. Things were going from dismal to more dismal; yet at the same time, the patients and staff were demanding more.

Jerry was hardly back in his office when the press called. It was a reporter from the local television station this time, presumably wanting his comments on the previous day's closure. He agreed to take the call. He responded smoothly and couldn't help but feel slightly pleased as the words tumbled from his mouth, but then the reporter blindsided him.

"So what's your response to the picketers?"

Jerry went to his window and scanned the street. "Well, as always, I prefer not to comment until I've had time to consider the issues from all sides. It is always a bit of a disappointment when a compromise can't be reached without moving an agenda out into a public forum." He could feel the perspiration beading on his forehead. "Let's just say that I have no comment for now."

He dropped the receiver even as he heard the reporter speaking and pulled out a handkerchief to wipe his brow. "Deborah," he bellowed, "the reporter said someone was picketing. Find out who it is and what they want. And don't let me talk to anymore reporters, will you? If anyone else calls, route them to Public Relations."

Ann, the new manager of the Emergency department, appeared in the outer office. Jerry could hear her addressing Deborah. "I need to talk to Jerry about a man who is picketing outside the entrance."

"Come in, I just got a call from a reporter. What's going on?" Jerry said, holding his door open.

"A man came to the emergency room seeking pain drugs the other night. It was the third time this week and the ER doctor wouldn't give him anything. We'd gotten word that on the other nights he was going to Dover to St. Mary's and doing the same thing. We offered to help him get a regular doctor so he could get the help he needs. One of the nurses even suggested rehab, but he just got mad. Now he's got a sign and he's walking up and down the sidewalk outside the ER. It says 'Peaceful Valley Memorial doesn't care about people in pain.' Can we call the police and have him removed? He's scaring the patients who really need us." Ann explained.

"Is he right outside the door?"

"No," she said, "he's on the sidewalk by the street."

Jerry shook his head. "Then we can't do a thing and he knows it. As long as he's not impeding traffic or the flow of the pedestrians, he's within his rights of free speech."

"We have to do something."

"Ignore him. That's the best thing we can do. And don't talk to any reporters."

Ann looked ready to cry. "This is my first month on the job. The EMTs [emergency medical technicians] are mad at the nurses, two night nurses just resigned, and now we have a picketer."

"Welcome to the world of healthcare," he tried to joke. "Sounds like you've got plenty to worry about. Don't waste time on the things you can't do anything about." He patted her shoulder and directed her toward the door.

It was after 2:00 P.M. before Jerry had a chance to think about lunch. The cafeteria hot line was closed and he was reduced to getting a hot dog. With all the care his wife took to feed him healthy meals and keep his cholesterol down, he couldn't help but feel guilty.

"It's better if you chew." It was Georgia. "Do you know that hot dogs are the most common cause of choking in children? Because they take big bites and forget to chew. Are you on your way to safety committee? I'll walk with you and fill you in on something. It might save you from another meeting."

"Bless you, Georgia."

She laughed. "You may take that blessing right back when you hear what I have to say. Did you hear about the man up on Six West? He was in for treatment of endocarditis and got up during the night and fell. He cracked his head on a chair in the room and had to have a CT scan and a couple of stitches in his forehead."

"Was this about two months ago?" Jerry asked.

"Yes."

"And I suppose you're telling me that we've heard from his lawyer."

"Good guess," she said.

"Was it our fault?"

Georgia shook her head. "He was ambulatory, no history of falls or stroke, no identified risks. The night nurse had just been in to check on him and said he was alert and watching TV. So he must have gotten up to go to the bathroom and tripped over his own feet."

"Think the lawyer is on a fishing expedition?"

Georgia shrugged. "More than likely, but you know how it is. If you look hard enough."

They stopped outside the conference room. "Any more good news before we go in?" Jerry asked.

"No, but then this meeting is always full of surprises."

Georgia was right, of course. Not only was there a surprise, but it was an expensive one. The meeting started with the usual chitchat, reports from the ER, the results of the fire inspector's visit, a report from the head of Security, a discussion about the oxygen shutoff valves and the negative pressure room for patients needing special respiratory isolation. Then talk turned to employee needlesticks and the Occupational Safety and Health Administration's (OSHA) mandate that the hospital convert to a needleless system of intravenous therapy. It would cost $23,000 annually.

"We've already converted to IV needles that retract after they're used," Joe from Materiels was saying. "We did that about three years ago and it cost us about $35,000 per year, two and a half times what we were paying. Now we're looking at changing to IV lines that have special ports that don't accept needles. All the injectable pharmacy medications will have to be converted so the drugs can be administered directly through the ports without a needle. The final phase will be getting syringes for intramuscular injections that retract after the needle is removed from the patient. All totaled it should run an additional $23,000 a year."

"Can some of it be held off until the next fiscal year?" Jerry asked.

Joe nodded. "We can, as long as OSHA believes that we're making a good-faith effort to convert to all safety products."

"And if they don't?" asked Georgia.

"Then they fine us."

Jerry looked around the table. "What's next?"

"Preparation for a biological terrorist attack," responded Kevin, the safety officer. "Smallpox vaccines."

The rest of the meeting was devoted to disasters. By the time Jerry returned to his office, he was thinking anxiously of his daughter, who worked in New York City. He wished she would consider moving closer to home.

Mary was waiting in the outer office. He had forgotten that they had a meeting scheduled. "Just let me get a drink, Mary," he said to stall for time. "Can I get you something?"

She shook her head. "I've asked Hillary to join us. I'll wait for her."

Mary and Hillary wasted no time getting to the point. "We felt we couldn't bring this up in a group meeting, Jerry, but it's too important to ignore. We've got some real issues in Nursing and if we don't attend to them now, we could be in a much worse state soon. Why don't you start, Hillary," Mary said.

"We're looking at a 15 percent vacancy rate in Nursing, Jerry. The worst shift, of course, is nights. We can hardly get them trained before they move on. St. Mary's is offering a sign-on bonus of $3,000 for any night nurse and requiring them to stay only six months to get it. And it's only a forty-five minute drive, so the incentive is pretty attractive. The nurses are complaining about being pulled by the nursing shift managers to cover other areas and the staff is really starting to feel the crunch."

"Last week we had four nurses on Three West, to give care to twenty-eight patients. The nurses feel like it isn't safe, and they're right," Mary added.

"And then of course there's the threat of a union. If we let things go too far, they'll get a foothold here."

Jerry folded his hands on the table. "I know you heard the same message I heard from Howard this morning."

"We did," Mary agreed, "but patients come to a hospital for nursing care. Without them, there is no hospital."

"I'm suggesting incentives," Hillary said, "for working extra shifts, for being pulled to other units, and a 6 percent pay raise across the board, effective immediately."

Jerry sucked in his breath. "Ouch! That will be pretty costly, won't it?"

"All totaled, I would guess in the hundred-thousand-dollar range, but we have to retain the nurses we have. The constant turnover will cost us much more in the long run," Hillary responded.

"There must be something other than money," Jerry exclaimed.

"There is," agreed Mary. "They want a voice. They want decisions about how care is given to be made by clinical people. Magnet status. You've heard of it, haven't you? Hospitals that give nurses more self-governance, give them the authority to reorganize the way they give care so that it is both the most efficient and of the highest quality."

They continued talking and ended with Jerry agreeing that they needed to make a presentation at the next board meeting, that he couldn't authorize that kind of expenditure alone.

As they adjourned, Jerry rose from his chair. "I guess we don't have to ask ourselves why we aren't making any money."

It was nearly 8:00 when Jerry left his office that night. He had stayed to answer the thank-you letters from the patients. Deborah had added one to the pile before she left, from a new father who had witnessed his wife going through a difficult delivery. He said that what the nurses and doctor had done was nothing short of a miracle. He savored that one, read it twice. As he turned to switch off the lights, he spied his jacket, still folded neatly over the chair where he had placed it when he entered. He never had had time to put it on. He picked it up and put it over his arm out of habit. Tomorrow, he thought, he might like to carry the navy jacket.

CHAPTER FOUR
Hospital Economics
HOW NURSES WERE LOST

If nurses are as dissatisfied as they reported in the ANA survey and if their working conditions have deteriorated so significantly that they fear they are not giving good quality care, why is it that the Jerry Standhills of the world initially failed to notice? The nurses who are giving daily care to patients may think that they were ignored because, as many expressed in the survey, the "suits" at the top just didn't care. The likelier answer, however, is that hospital administrators didn't fully understand the nature of the problem.

My own story may serve as an illustration. In 1985 I was working as an RN on a medical-surgical unit. One weekend, due to unscheduled staff absences resulting from a snowstorm, I was assigned ten patients to care for. At the start of the shift, I felt panicky, fearing that I just couldn't physically attend to ten patients in an eight-hour shift. I quickly explained to the three patients who were nearly ready for discharge and able to perform their own basic daily care that we were short-staffed and that I would check back with them as often as I could. I reminded them to use the nurse call button if they needed something and didn't see me. To another patient who was awaiting surgery, and also capable of performing most of his own care, I repeated the same message, which left me just about enough time to adequately care for the remaining six patients. I was carried through the shift by adrenaline (certainly there was no time for lunch) and when it was over, I was exhausted but satisfied with a job well done. I was glad to get back to my usual seven patients the next day. But in retrospect, I felt good about the previous day's challenge. In 1986 I took a position in an outpatient infusion center, but continued to work extra shifts as needed on the inpatient units. If there was a change in the patient population and the resulting workload, I didn't really notice it. By the early 1990s the duties of my primary job prevented me from doing extra shifts in the hospital and it wasn't until the late 1990s that I returned as a relief weekend-shift supervisor. I found a very different landscape than the one I had so recently left. As the shift supervisor, it was my job to ensure that each unit had adequate staffing and to float staff from a unit that had more than enough nurses to units that were short. What I discovered when I made rounds to each unit was that there was a big gap between what I thought was adequate staffing and what the nurses on duty thought was adequate! And my direct experience as a staff nurse had come from only a few years earlier. For hospital CEOs all over the country, especially those with no clinical background, the noise coming from the nursing units must have been even more baffling. What the nurses doing the work understood and others didn't was that the nature of their work had changed dramatically in a very short period of time.

A BRIEF HISTORY OF HEALTHCARE

To understand what happened and why it had such a powerful impact, it is necessary to review a short history of American healthcare. Perhaps a part of the answer lies in the alphabet soup of acronyms through which hospital administrators have had to wade in the last two decades. HMO, DRG, PPS, JCAHO, HCFA, CMS, APC and HIPAA are just a few of the letter groupings that need to be thoroughly understood to operate a hospital in the new millennium. Gone are the Marcus Welby days when physicians were presumed to be kindly, wise, courageous men and when hospitals were amply staffed with nurses who understood "their place," gliding through the halls in soft white shoes and even whiter uniforms with their hair demurely covered by their nursing caps. It is no longer possible to run a hospital fueled only by an administrator's goodwill and political savvy. Hospital CEOs hold advanced degrees in hospital administration and are assisted by experts in planning, development, human resources, and finance. Together they navigate an ever-changing minefield of physician, staff, and patient demands in the face of shrinking economic returns and burgeoning costs.

During the 1950s, the 1960s, and even into the 1970s, American hospitals enjoyed a kind of golden age—at least from an administrator's point of view—starting with the widespread use of penicillins. Patients who were dying of infections, to whom physicians and nurses had previously been able to offer only kindness and comfort, suddenly found themselves cured. A nurse who trained in the early 1950s told of treating hospital patients admitted with pneumonia. "You hated to see them come in. We'd set up those awful oxygen tents. They were cumbersome and humid and gave the patients claustrophobia. You knew just by looking at them that most of them weren't going to make it. It was awful. And then came penicillin and people started getting better. It was like a miracle." That miracle served to alter the public image of physicians. They were no longer just kindly faced gentlemen dispensing warmth, but genuine healers, men who had the power to save lives. And hospitals were no longer frightening places that swallowed up loved ones, but places that people left feeling better than when they entered.

But antibiotics were only the beginning. What followed were better insulins for diabetes and cardiac drugs to counter arrhythmias or reduce blood pressure. Simple X rays spawned CT (computed tomography) scans, MRIs (magnetic resonance imaging), and ultrasounds. And all of it came at a price. Hospital administrators spent money to acquire the latest technology and drugs and passed on the cost to consumers. Suddenly Americans needed health insurance for hospitalizations. In 1965 President Johnson introduced Medicare and Medicaid programs to ensure that the elderly and the poor were able to receive healthcare.

A System of Cost Reimbursement

For a couple of decades, cost remained a nonissue to hospital administrators. They operated under a cost reimbursement or fee-for-service model. When a patient entered the hospital, the services they received—including drugs, diagnostic tests, surgical procedures, and supplies—were recorded and tallied. The room charge was determined separately based on hospital overhead. The bill that was ultimately presented to the patient and/or the insurer represented the sum of the room charge plus the itemized services. Charges were rarely challenged by the payors. Initially, even Medicare and Medicaid reimbursed according to the invoices received. But as healthcare became more complex, the fee-for-service system proved too simple to respond to the challenges. Rather than encourage cost containment, it seemed to reward waste. For example, a hospital that acquired a new CT scanner under the fee-for-service system might be tempted to encourage physician overusage so the equipment's cost could more quickly be recovered. At the same time, hospitals were free to pass on their inefficiencies to the patients. A hospital that staffed according to need and was judicious in its use of supplies charged less and received less, while one that was extravagant with staff and wasteful of supplies simply charged— and received—higher fees. Hospitals weren't likely to encourage their physicians to discharge patients in a timely manner. If a physician wished his patient to remain in the hospital merely for a few days of rest, the hospital was reimbursed regardless of need. Of course, the vast majority of physicians and hospital administrators strove to offer the highest quality care at the most reasonable price, but the flaws in the system began to show.

Healthcare costs rose rapidly throughout the 1960s. Medicare, which insures about 99 percent of the elderly population, is administered federally by CMS (formerly the Health Care Finance Administration, or HCFA), and accounts for about a third of all inpatient hospital stays. In most states, Medicaid hospital stays run a close second. After the programs were introduced, they began absorbing more and more medical costs. Within a few years of their inception, the amount of money invested by the federal government into Medicare programs nearly doubled and less than a decade later the amount doubled again. To curb the rising costs without cutting the benefits to the elderly, disabled, and poor, a radical overhaul of the system was needed.

Prospective Payment Systems and DRGs

In the 1970s some states, including New York, were experimenting with a rate-setting system whereby hospitals were paid a preset fee per patient day. If a patient entered a hospital, the facility was paid a certain rate per day regardless of the services used. Since the rates were announced at the beginning of the year, the plan was called a prospective payment system (PPS). Capping the rate gave hospitals an incentive to reduce or control their costs and knowing the rate ahead of time gave the institutions a better opportunity to budget accordingly. It didn't work equally well for all hospitals, however. The hospitals that served sicker patients and handled more complex treatments were penalized, since their patients required more costly services. Still it was seen as a successful enough concept that by 1983, Medicare was introducing its own PPS, called diagnosis related groupings (DRGs). Upon admission to a hospital, the patients were categorized into one of 470 different treatment/illness groups and hospitals were paid a set rate according to the severity of illness.

Though not a perfect system, Medicare's DRG rate setting did have the desired effect. The number of hospital stays paid by Medicare declined in the first year, as did the average length of stay. Most importantly, it took a bite out of the hospital cost inflation rate, which had been running in the double digits. As Medicare moved to DRGs, the other major insurers soon followed suit in a modified version.

What was good for the economy, however, was not necessarily good for nursing. Under the DRG system, hospitals were encouraged to cut costs—including staffing, pay raises, and the purchase of new equipment—to maintain a profit. (Although the majority of hospitals are still nonprofit, they need to maintain at least a small profit margin to cover operating expenses, the replacement of worn equipment, unexpected costs, or reimbursement cuts.) Urban hospitals serving a higher proportion of patients insured by Medicaid were hit even harder. Medicaid is paid only partly with federal funds. The remaining dollars come from the individual states that administer the programs, which often reimburse at a much lower level. The irony is that the urban hospitals with large trauma centers that may need the highest ratio of nurses to patients are the ones with the greatest incentive to cut staffing.

Managed Care

Health maintenance organizations (HMOs) added a whole new flavor to the healthcare menu in the late 1980s. Like Medicare's DRGs, the intent of HMOs is cost containment. An HMO can appear in different models with varying degrees of control over the healthcare offered. In the most rigid model, the HMO actually employs the physicians and may even own its own facilities. Membership is sold, often to big employers, at a reduced cost and all members are required to receive their healthcare from the HMO physicians at designated facilities. In that instance, the HMO is a major competitor to existing hospitals.

Even in lesser controlled models, however, managed care was perceived as a threat to hospitals and healthcare systems. If a managed care organization did not own its own facilities, it could still dictate the facilities the consumer used. It sold a service to employers, promising that it could contain costs for healthcare benefits for their employees. If the pitch was good and enough memberships were sold, it wielded a great deal of economic power. Enrollees were allowed to use only the physicians and facilities that the HMO designated or they had to pay out of their own pocket. That put the HMO in a strong negotiating position with area hospitals and physicians. Providers that refused to accept the organization's (cut) rates would be effectively frozen out from access to any of its enrollees. And of course, since the managed care organizations needed to make profits to survive, they added one more cut to an already shrinking pie. For instance, suppose healthcare monies were represented by one dollar, and thirty cents of that dollar went to physicians and seventy cents went to hospitals. Out of the hospital's seventy cents, forty cents might be spent on equipment and facility overhead, and twenty-five cents on operations, including employee pay and benefits. That leaves five cents as a narrow profit margin. With the addition of managed care, the dollar had not grown, costs for the hospital remained the same, but now three cents had to go to the managed care administrative organization for brokering the agreement. Thus, the prospect of managed care incited anxiety for hospital CEOs.

Ambulatory Payment Classifications

Since insurers, led by Medicare, were actively discouraging inpatient hospital admissions by the end of the 1980s, hospitals had to find a way to recoup some of their losses. Industry experts advised hospitals to reduce their number of inpatient beds and instead invest in outpatient facilities. Many of them did, at a cost of millions of dollars. But as the new millennium began, CMS cut reimbursements to home care agencies for nursing, physical therapy, and healthcare aide services. At the same time, they announced their plan for ambulatory payment classifications (APCs) as a means of controlling payments for other outpatient care that was provided by a facility. For some services, such as outpatient cancer care, the impact has proven significant. For example, brachytherapy is a means of inserting radioactive sources directly into the area of the body in which a tumor lies, and either removing the source after a prescribed time period or leaving it in place if the source is less radioactive. It has been a useful treatment option for prostate cancer and, more recently, for breast cancer. In the fall of 2002, CMS announced its APC listing for 2003. It included a bundling of several of the separate brachytherapy charges into one APC, effectively reducing reimbursement by approximately 40 percent. Medical oncology also stood to take a sizable hit as some high-cost chemotherapeutic agents and the antiemetic (antinausea) drugs given with them to control the side effects were bundled into one chemotherapy administration APC. The choice of drugs was still up to the physicians, of course, but the reimbursement rate would be the same regardless of the cost—discouraging the use of the newer, high-cost drugs.

Ironically, in 2003, not only is the outpatient profit margin shrinking, but with a number of hospitals going under in the 1990s, some of the urban hospitals that managed to remain in business suddenly find that they don't have enough inpatient beds to meet their city's need.

QUALITY AND ACCREDITATION

Quality, which was once just considered a natural part of delivering healthcare, has taken on its own identity in the last decade. In 1951 the Joint Commission on Accreditation of Hospitals (JCAH) was established by a group of physicians as an offshoot of the American College of Surgeons. By 1953 the JCAH was quietly publishing standards and conducting accreditation surveys for hospitals; and in 1964 it began charging for its visits. Many hospitals voluntarily sought the accreditation of the JCAH, grateful for a means of measuring the quality of care they gave, but the federal government lent the surveys real weight by attaching payments to accreditation. The Social Security Amendments of 1965 included a stipulation that only accredited hospitals could participate in the Medicare and Medicaid programs. Over the decades that followed, the JCAH expanded its role to long-term care facilities, managed-care organizations, laboratories, home-care organizations, and psychiatric facilities, to name a few. To accommodate the expansion, it changed its name to the Joint Commission on Accreditation of Healthcare Organizations and focused on performance-based standards, emphasizing important patient safety issues that previously had not been addressed.

The accreditation process has undoubtedly enhanced the safety and quality of care for patients. Standardization of care allows for collection and comparison of data, continuing improvements, and oversight of an extremely complex field with a high potential for causing harm along with healing, but it is not without both direct and indirect costs for a hospital. Accreditation surveys are conducted at least every three years—for hospital laboratories, every two years. The survey cost averages about $20,000, according to JCAHO sources, but when the cost of compliance is factored in, the true fiscal impact on an organization grows substantially. A comprehensive manual from the JCAHO that includes hospital standards, scoring, and examples of compliance runs more than one thousand pages. The standards are fluid, constantly changing to reflect current quality concerns and trends in medicine. A healthcare organization needs a full-time high-functioning employee to oversee the JCAHO regulations and requires untold hours from nursing administrators, pharmacists, infection control specialists, facility managers, and medical directors to ensure that all staff members are in compliance with the regulations. Savvy organizations also pay for mock surveys on their off years to ensure that they are meeting the newest standards. The regulation of quality—and the documentation necessary to prove it—has required an increasingly large commitment of time and money by healthcare institutions.

At the same time, the increasingly painstaking accreditation surveys have impacted nurse satisfaction. As one frustrated nurse responded in a questionnaire, "If we didn't have to spend so much time trying to prove we *gave* good care, we'd have more time *for* good care."

THE COST OF TECHNOLOGY

Technology has significantly altered the face of healthcare over the last decades. Americans have access to some of the most advanced technology in the world, but the changes are coming so quickly it is hard for a hospital and the staff who use the technology to keep up. Only twenty years ago, hospital equipment was often assigned a ten-year life expectancy and could be depreciated over that time. Depreciation as an accounting function helped reduce the impact of a large expenditure of funds by spreading it over the useful life of the item. New technology has not only dramatically increased in price, but its depreciation period has shortened due to rapid advances. A manager of a medical imaging department told me that he had no sooner purchased and installed a CT scanner with a $2-million price tag, than it became obsolete. And one new product does not necessarily eliminate the need for the other. It simply enhances capability. Again, medical imaging is a good example. The introduction of the CT scanner did not replace the necessity or usefulness of simple X rays. It merely added a new dimension in diagnostic testing, just as the MRI did not decrease the need for the CT scanner and the positive emitting tomography (PET) scanner did not replace the MRI. Having expensive equipment does not necessarily mean a facility's income will increase. Diagnostic testing done during an inpatient stay is not reimbursed separately by insurers such as Medicare and Medicaid. It is simply rolled into their DRG reimbursement as part of the cost of giving care. In other words, a certain amount of money is paid to a hospital based on a patient's diagnosis and the care that is expected for that particular illness. An extra fee is not collected just because expensive equipment is used for a diagnostic test.

PHARMACEUTICALS

For hospitals, pharmaceutical development is another double-edged sword. On the one hand, new medications may offer great promise for previously incurable conditions or comfort where previously there was only misery. On the other hand, the price of the new therapies and the complexity of their administration may substantially add to a hospital's cost of doing business without a corresponding means of increasing reimbursements.

Return again to medical oncology (the treatment of cancer by systemic chemotherapy or immunotherapy). Twenty years ago, patients who received chemotherapy with high emetic (vomiting) probability had to face difficult choices about the value of treatment, deciding if the potential cure was worth the misery of the extensive nausea and vomiting it caused. The older antinausea medications simply could not counter the side effects of some chemotherapeutic regimens. Then, in the 1990s, ondansetron and granisetron appeared on the market. Suddenly patients who once might have suffered days of vomiting were undergoing chemotherapy treatments with their nausea largely controlled. Yet despite such improvements and the increased cure potential, some chemotherapy threatened patients' lives because the dosages killed not only the cancer but also the infection-fighting white blood cells. As a result, even a simple cold could progress to something more dangerous in a patient's compromised immune system. The risk made proper dosing a difficult call for physicians, but in the 1990s, about the same time that the new class of antiemetics was introduced, new drugs emerged as alternatives to dose reduction. Colony stimulators encouraged growth of white cells, enabling patients to better tolerate the negative effects of higher-dose chemotherapy. For the patients receiving the drugs and the doctors and nurses administering them, the result was undeniably beneficial. The cost, however, was prohibitive. For the antiemetics, the cost could be ten times the cost of the older drugs. And the colony-stimulating factors could be hundreds of dollars per dose. Again, without the capability of passing on the increased costs to the patient or insurance company, the impact on the hospital for an inpatient stay that included chemotherapy could be significant.

Janet Silvester, MBA, RPh, director of the pharmacy at a nonprofit community hospital, wonders how larger urban hospitals with sicker populations are able to manage with the 2003 CMS rate changes for medications. Using as an example a new category of medication that has been shown to be effective against sepsis (an uncommon but often fatal massive infection), Silvester points out that for Medicare patients, "Hospitals get paid less than it costs to purchase the drug. Then the drug has to be reconstituted (prepared for administration) under a special laminar flow hood, so added to the expense of drug acquisition is the cost of the hood, the personnel, and supplies. How can a hospital do that and stay in business?" For some medications, hospitals can choose to discourage their use by not including them in the pharmacy inventory of drugs, but not including a therapy that has demonstrated such a clear advantage in saving lives would be unconscionable. For those who are fiscally responsible to the hospital, however, it is another cost that somehow needs to be accounted for.

PREVENTION OF MEDICAL ERRORS

Preventable medical errors are responsible for more deaths per year than auto accidents, according to a 1999 report by the Institute of Medicine, a private, nonprofit organization that provides health policy advice.[1] Many of those errors revolve around the administration of medication, a function largely relegated to nurses. With the growth in new drugs and their specific uses for a small range of symptoms, the five "rights" taught in nursing school—right patient, right drug, right dose, right route, and right time—increases in importance. An error of omission or delivering the wrong medication to a patient can have catastrophic results. Yet with all other aspects of patient care increasing in complexity at the same time, the possibility of error is growing rather than shrinking. A pharmacist remarked to me that she "didn't know how the nurses can keep up with all the new drugs and their indications. It's hard for us as pharmacists and that's all we do, but a nurse has to be concerned with all other elements of a patient's care and then give the medications on top of it." During the 1960s and 1970s, new drugs came out at a rate of about fifteen to twenty drugs a year, giving nurses time to learn their indications and expected side effects. Now the Food and Drug Administration approves as many as fifty new drugs per year,[2] making it nearly impossible for nurses to familiarize themselves with the particular indications of their administration.

An electronic means of double-checking such as the bar coding of patient medication doses can help reduce medication errors. After the physician writes an order, it can be entered into a computer system that produces bar-coded labels. A pharmacy robot is referred by the bar code to the correct drug at the correct dose and it packages the medication accordingly. Prior to administration, the nurse uses a bar-code reader to double-check that the medication she is about to give matches the wrist band of the patient to whom it is being delivered, ensuring that the right drug at the right dose is being delivered to the right patient.

Another means of eliminating medication error is by ridding the system of interpretation by the nurse or pharmacy technician who has to decipher the physician's handwriting and instead allowing the physicians to enter their medication orders directly into the pharmacy computer. For nurses, a computerized clinical documentation system that has prompts for certain vital assessment data can both shorten charting time and enhance communication to other members of the healthcare team. Information can be entered via a handheld device at the bedside or a mobile station just outside a patient's door. This kind of comprehensive software system streamlines all aspects of patient care, including accurate billing, but it comes with a multimillion-dollar price tag.

Once again, hospital administrators are faced with difficult choices. Without the ability to pass on the cost to the consumer, the purchase of the software may adversely affect the hospital's ability to increase the nurse-to-patient ratio (another patient care quality issue) and maintain competitive wages for their employees.

HEALTH INSURANCE PORTABILITY AND ACCOUNTABILITY ACT

A previously unheard-of acronym that has now become part of the hospital vernacular is HIPAA, referring to the 1996 Health Insurance Portability and Accountability Act, the federal government's mandate to protect patients' medical information from misuse and inappropriate disclosure. Volumes of health information are compiled daily and stored in paper files as well as in huge computer databanks. Data are transported by mail, by fax, and across the Internet on "protected" systems, but personal health information is a sensitive issue. Not only is simple privacy an important right, but health information has been used illegally by employers, prospective employers, and insurers to discriminate against people with certain illnesses or disabilities. For many reasons, the awareness of and need for confidentiality of personal medical information has grown. A physician can now view the lab results of her patient from any remote designated station, which enhances her ability to treat in a timely fashion, but if physicians or other caregivers can access the data with a few keystrokes, how easily can the confidentiality of records be compromised?

When HIPAA was passed in 1996, it gave Congress three years to pass further legislation that would protect the privacy of health information. Since Congress failed to do so in the allotted time, the responsibility fell to the Department of Health and Human Services (DHHS). The proposed HIPAA regulations as presented by the DHHS have different parts, but the privacy standards that became effective April 14, 2003, are currently having the greatest impact on healthcare institutions. The regulations outline the actions that hospitals and other healthcare providers are expected to take to ensure the privacy of a patient's protected health information (PHI), including the establishment of a written notice of privacy practices and a mechanism for distribution/publication. They also mandate designating an organizational official who will accept responsibility for administration of the safeguards, establish the procedures for allowing individuals to make complaints about privacy issues, and punish the violators. Policies and procedures must be established to handle patient requests for their health information and to ensure "minimum necessary information" is communicated when sharing a patient's PHI with other entities (physicians, insurers, and other members of the healthcare team) for purposes of treatment, payment, or healthcare operations. And once all the policies, procedures, safeguards, and penalties have been established, an organization-wide training program has to be instituted—and incorporated into the orientation programs of all new employees. And, since the federal HIPAA regulations are meant to be only an adjunct to state laws, not to supercede them if the state laws are stricter, there must be a comparison done between state and federal laws to ensure appropriate compliance.

A director of nursing told me that "it's not just HIPAA by itself. It's trying to figure out what to do when regulations appear to be in conflict. If HIPAA says one thing and JCAHO says another, and the state yet another, which takes precedence?"

Administratively, the investment of time and money related to HIPAA alone is immense. The interpretation and implementation of the regulations and the education of staff requires input from a whole team of personnel, from nurses to administrators to financial staff to medical records staff. Documentation of the program alone may necessitate the addition of new personnel to the payroll. And continuing review of policy prior to implementation may also involve legal counsel, adding further to costs.

THE COST OF LITIGATION

Few would argue that if human error causes another person significant harm, some compensation should be provided. Everyone has heard reports of a death caused by medical error, a wrong limb amputated, or some other egregious act performed on an unsuspecting patient. In legal terms, that constitutes negligence and is the basis for compensatory awards. The real headache lies in finding a fair system for determining which cases merit compensation and their respective amounts. Currently, the only certain means the American public has of seeking compensation for an injury caused by a healthcare provider is by litigation. One of the problems with lawsuits is that they come after the fact, sometimes several years later (depending on the state's statute of limitations), when there is no longer any means of correcting a genuine or perceived wrong. Even if a financial settlement is not the plaintiff's ultimate goal, at that point in time it is difficult to find any alternative means of settling a dispute. As the only avenue for settlement of disputes, the number of lawsuits has increased along with the amount of the awards, necessitating that hospitals employ risk managers and enlarge their budgets to include legal consultations and increased insurance premiums. Importantly, whether a lawsuit brought against a hospital is valid or not, the institution still has to pay to defend itself, and sometimes the legal fees incurred in winning are greater than the penalty for losing.

While the financial cost is substantial, the intangible costs are at least as great a concern. The prevalence of litigation coupled with publicity surrounding medical errors has promoted an adversarial relationship between the healthcare provider and the recipient, from which neither benefits. An atmosphere of general distrust doesn't inspire the nurse to give the best care, nor does it actively promote patient healing. The issue is discussed further in chapter 11, but merits mention here as one more worrisome factor competing with the nursing crisis for the attention of hospital administrators.

THE EFFECT ON NURSES

In light of the pressures coming from multiple arenas, it is not difficult to understand how hospital administrators could have been temporarily blinded to the plight of the nurses. Yet in hindsight, it is apparent that the same changes capturing the attention of administrators were also influencing the nurses' daily workload.

Let's go back to the day in 1985 when I had to care for ten patients. Three were nearing discharge and one was a patient admitted prior to surgery. None of the four had intravenous therapy and all four were ambulatory (able to move about unassisted). Those patients would not be in a hospital today. No insurer would pay for their stay. When I was working on that unit, I would expect about three of seven patients to have an IV in their arm. Their IVs ran by gravity and I would set the proper rate by counting the drips flowing from the IV bag. Most of the medications were oral, in the form of pills. On the same unit now, at least seven of eight patients have an IV, some of which are going through a simple intravenous catheter in the arm, while others are going through a special line into a large central vein that have very strict guidelines for care due to the risk of transmitting bacteria and causing a serious infection very quickly. Many of the patients' medications are given via IV. Few if any IVs run by simple gravity, but instead run through pumps that control their rates and must be programmed carefully by the nurse. Some have a secondary line piggybacked into the first, often with a patient-controlled analgesia pump attached so that patients can administer their own pain medication. This pump also has to be carefully regulated and monitored to avoid overmedicating a patient with dangerous narcotics. But the IVs are only one small aspect of nursing care. The same patients likely have surgical wounds that require special care, are unable to walk without assistance, and may be in altered mental states that require close monitoring to prevent accidental self-injury. They may require oxygen therapy and multiple tests and procedures that necessitate transporting them to other units. They may need special tube feedings and Foley catheters to drain their urine. Importantly, they are likely also to be in need of intensive teaching before they leave the hospital so they can care for themselves at home. In other words, as stays in the hospital have shortened, the patients who are there tend to be sicker and the work of the nurse is greatly intensified. Whereas only six of my ten patients in 1985 required substantive care, now every patient requires intense care and the increased knowledge and expertise to give it.

The shorter lengths of stay create another hidden addition to the workload. A patient census is taken at midnight. A given unit might have twenty-six patients. The next night at midnight, the census might be exactly the same, but unlike just a decade ago when most of the twenty-six were the same patients, in today's environment, ten may have been discharged and another ten admitted to take their place. For the nurse, this translates to the need for conducting complete new physical assessments and learning the new patients' medications, diagnoses, treatments, physical limitations, allergies, and so on, while the patients with whom the nurse has just become familiar are gone.

But it is not just a change in intensity of care that has impacted nurses. At the same time, regulatory agencies such as JCAHO have stepped up their surveillance on patient safety. While it is administrators who struggle to interpret the standards, it is the nurses who have to apply them correctly. Take the case of patient restraints as an example. At one time, if a patient was confused and pulling at vital postoperative tubes or drains or IV lines, a resourceful nurse may have applied a soft cotton restraint to the patient's wrist to prevent him from hurting himself. She checked him regularly during her rounds, but could attend to her other patients somewhat assured of that patient's safety. Currently, the regulations call for a nurse to call the doctor and get an order for restraints, but only after she has documented that she has exhausted all other possibilities, including distracting the patient's attention elsewhere, closer monitoring, or requesting that a family member sit with the patient. If a restraint order is received, documentation has to reflect that she continues to look for alternatives and that she checks the patient at least every two hours. That is, she cannot just check the patient; she has to make a notation in the patient's chart each time that she did so. The intention is a positive impact on patient safety, but without a significant reduction in the number of patients, the nurse's daily work is impossible to complete.

The time it took for hospital CEOs to recognize the nurses', dire circumstances—and not all have yet—may be perfectly understandable to some, but to nurses it may be hard to forgive. The nurses that responded to both the ANA and my own survey expressed a surprising amount of emotion. They felt betrayed. They had lost faith in their institutions and distrusted the motivations of those who manage the healthcare facilities. They still felt loyalty to the patients and the mission of their profession, but they no longer believed in their employers' mission. What can be done to regain their trust and the changes that need to take place in the workplace will be discussed in chapter 8, but first there is another important member of the healthcare team to consider.

What, if any, role do physicians play in the growing shortage of nurses? And if the shortage reaches critical proportions, how will it affect the work of physicians?

NOTES

1. William C. Richardson et al., "To Err Is Human: Building a Safer Health System," Institute of Medicine [online], www.iom.edu/includes/dbfile. asp?id=4117 [November 1999].

2. David Dranove, *The Economic Evolution of American Health Care: From Marcus Welby to Managed Care* (Princeton, N.J.: Princeton University Press, 2000), p. 14.

CHAPTER FIVE

Nurses and Doctors

W hat is it about doctors and nurses? Between individual members of both groups there are many friendships and obvious
indications of mutual appreciation and respect, but ask either about the
other as a group and the grumbling begins. Yet nurses and doctors are
both essential members of the same team, both working toward a
mutual goal of quality patient care. Perhaps the dissension occurs
because they don't always agree on the path for achieving their goal and
because they don't share a common style of communication.

Communication between doctors and nurses often begins with the
physician writing an order, the prescription for treatment and medication. The term itself sets up a potentially adversarial relationship from
the outset, as it implies one member of the team is superior to the
other, rather than that they simply perform different functions. In a
hospital, after the doctor visits a patient and writes orders, he leaves and
returns to his office practice. The nurse has no prescriptive powers,* but
is with the patient the other twenty-three and a half hours of the day,
constantly assessing the results of the prescribed course of treatment. If
the results aren't as anticipated, the nurse has to inform the doctor prior
to deviating from the prescribed plan. This is where the relationship can

---

*In many states, nurse practitioners have prescriptive rights, but they are rarely employed
on general nursing units.

really deteriorate. Just as not all nurses are equally competent at articulating a problem, not all physicians can tolerate an unwanted communication without blaming the messenger. A nurse inexperienced in communicating vital information might tell a doctor that "Mr. Jones is feeling faint. He looks like he's going bad." To a physician (a scientist), such a statement is meaningless. What looks? How are his vital signs? What does his lab work indicate? And if the nurse's insight proves predictive, it may only increase the physician's frustration as he has been given no concrete data with which he can assess and correct the problem, especially from a remote location such as his office or car. On the other hand, an experienced nurse may communicate all the right data and still receive a negative response such as yelling or castigation because she delivered news a physician did not want to hear.

Fairly or not, with the demand for nurses currently outstripping the supply, the nature of the relationship between doctor and nurse has begun receiving more attention as a possible factor in the decline of new recruits. And rare is the nurse who cannot relate at least one story of being publicly yelled at, hung up on, or otherwise made to feel small by a physician. A 1997 article in *Journal of Professional Nursing* said that more than 90 percent of nurses reported that they had witnessed at least one episode of verbal abuse by a physician in the previous year.[1] In the survey that I distributed at the INS nurses meeting, I included five questions that addressed the issue of respect in the workplace. Nurses were asked if they felt respected by the patients, other nurses, administrators, doctors, and other healthcare workers. Except for one negative vote, the nurses indicated that they always felt respected by the patients, and 92 percent indicated they felt respected by other nurses. Administrators were the least likely to be seen as respectful, but the doctors fared surprisingly poorly as well. Only 62 of the 132 responses to the question "Are you treated with respect by doctors?" were affirmative—less than half. Twenty-one were no and the remainder indicated "sometimes or usually." When asked the greatest source of frustration on the job, the most common responses included paperwork, not enough time with patients, and the lack of nonclinical administrators' understanding of the nurses' work, but nearly 6 percent cited physician blame and faultfinding as their number one complaint.

A survey conducted by VHA West Coast, a regional division of a nationwide network of community hospitals, and reported by Alan Rosenstein, MD, MBA, in the *American Journal of Nursing* considered the nurse-physician relationship in depth. The twelve hundred respondents included nurses, physicians, and executives from eighty-four different hospitals.[2] All three groups agreed that only a small percentage of physicians exhibited disruptive behavior, but the nurses and hospital executives reported that its impact was great, adversely affecting the attitude of nurses and other staff members who witnessed such behavior. Physicians indicated by their responses that they had neither observed the behavior as often nor thought that its impact on nurses' job satisfaction and morale was as great as the other two groups. More than 30 percent of the respondents, however, indicated that they personally knew of a nurse who had left the hospital as a direct result of physician behavior.[3]

Phone calls were cited by nurses in the VHA survey as one of the instances during which abusive behavior by physicians was most likely to occur. Other situations listed by the nurses included the questioning or clarification of physician orders, times when a physician perceived that his orders were not carried out in a timely or correct manner, and following a sudden change in the patients' status. The physicians' perspective was important in its distinctions. In the survey, physicians indicated that incorrectly carried-out orders were the primary cause of any ill behavior, followed by "ill-timed" phone calls and the nurses' need to question orders. They also noted that nurses often made calls to them without having all the pertinent data available.[4]

Regardless of the reason, it is clear that although disruptive behavior by physicians was once tolerated, nurses no longer find the behavior acceptable. They want to be treated respectfully, and with the nurse vacancy rate hovering around 13 percent nationally, their voice is beginning to have more clout. While the vast majority of physicians need no prodding, the repeat offenders may require more incentive to change than simply being told by nurses that their behavior is unacceptable. Hospital administrators who were reluctant to get involved in the past are now beginning to act. They have to fight to hold onto the staff they employ, and for many hospitals that has meant adopting a zero-tolerance policy of physician abuse. Nearly two-thirds of the respondents in the VHA survey indicated that their hospital had some such policy, although less than 50 percent indicated that they thought it was effective[5] due to lack of enforcement by hospital administrators. Since physicians are a hospital's main source of patient referrals and since they are not usually hospital employees, a hospital administrator may be reluctant or feel powerless to effect significant change in a physician's behavior.

Many physicians are surprised that a hospital would need such a policy, expressing disbelief that other doctors act in a manner that could be interpreted as abusive toward nurses. "Even if I disagree with a nurse's interpretation of a situation, I can't imagine screaming about it," a physician confided. "Doctors *need* nurses. It's just not smart to antagonize the people who help you give good care."

It is important to note again that most respondents of the VHA survey agreed that only 2 to 5 percent of the physicians acted in a questionable manner, which is to say that 95 to 98 percent do not. But the fact that it is being discussed and studied may open the way to another dialogue, that of the nurse's desire for increased autonomy. Since they are often at the point of care and the physician is not, nurses want some power to effect treatment changes they feel are necessary without waiting for an order from a physician who may be several blocks or even miles away in his office.

"Why do the best nurses go into administrative positions? I don't understand why hospitals let good nurses move away from the bedside."

I always smile when doctors ask me that question because I understand the kindness of their intent. And I'm pleased with the implication that they consider me a good nurse, but I am surprised that they don't know the answer. In a word, it is autonomy, the opportunity to use my judgment to make decisions and assume responsibility when the result is not what I had planned.

In most hospitals, nurses are the primary caregivers. Physicians visit patients in the hospital for minutes a day, while nurses staff the same hospital twenty-four hours a day, seven days a week. When a patient needs help, it is the nurse that he calls. (In teaching institutions, residents and interns are available as well.) Yet depending on the situation and the physician involved, few decisions can be made without the doctor's assent. Complicating the situation is that nurses on any given unit may have to interact with fifty or more different doctors and each doctor might have his own rules about what nurses are allowed to do without an order.

Clearly, of course, nurses can direct daily care. While treatments and medications are ordered by the physicians, how they are delivered is generally left up to the nurse. Much of the instruction that is given when a patient is discharged is conducted by the nurse. It is the nurse who performs regular assessments and monitors patients' conditions around the clock and whose actions serve to prevent complications following surgery or other invasive procedures. Most of these interventions are not dictated by physicians, but are determined by the nurse's judgment.

Between the doctor and nurse, however, there is a lot of gray area. One doctor may trust a nurse to make decisions about simple medications (such as antacids for indigestion, acetaminophen for headaches, or laxatives for constipation) and let him know what was done after the fact. Another physician may not want the nurse to so much as change a saturated dressing over a wound unless authorization is sought. And it may be that the same doctor will not allow two different nurses an equal amount of leeway. One example of an area where nurses and doctors often disagree is the point at which a patient's code status should be obtained. The code status refers to the type and limit of resuscitation efforts a patient desires if his heart stops beating and/or he stops breathing. Nurses often want the information before physicians feel it is necessary and as the group charged with being the patients' advocates, they feel it's important to give the patient the opportunity to express their wishes. However, for the most part, physicians consider this to be a subject broached only by the physician. Some doctors feel that by asking a hospitalized patient about their resuscitation preference, they could cause undue anxiety. The doctors may also fear that a "no code" status will cause the nurses to be less diligent in their care. The nurses, on the other hand, who are at the bedside, are the initiators of a code if some unforeseen event occurs and would like to know whether the patient wants everything possible done (and does he understand what "everything" means?) or wants to go peacefully. Obviously, it remains a point of contention.

Complicating the issue of distribution of power is that physicians, most of whom entered medical school with a reasonable expectation of the freedom to use their medical judgment to prescribe a course of treatment for their patients, are finding their independence squeezed at every turn. Managed care now often dictates what can be done in the way of both diagnostic tests and treatment by stating what will and will not be paid for. And many doctors are retreating into multiphysician partnerships that further reduce their autonomy because the cost of operating a physician practice has become prohibitive. With nurses wanting more control, the physicians are being asked to give up even more. From the nurse's perspective, a more collegial approach to caring for the patients will benefit everyone, but it is not hard to see why the concept might meet with some resistance from physicians who are taught to view themselves as the primary providers of care. The point of discussion, however, is finding solutions to the nursing shortage, and it is apparent that the doctor plays a direct role in the nurse's relative job satisfaction.

Dorothy, who was mentioned in an earlier chapter as a person who chose nursing at a time when limited options were available to women, was surprised when one of her daughters chose to become a nurse as well. I interviewed her daughter, Mina Ford, and asked what led to her choice. She said that when she graduated from high school, it had been the furthest thing from her mind. "After watching how hard my mother worked all those years, I thought I'd rather be anything than a nurse." But after completing four years of college, she began working in a physician's office when she couldn't immediately find employment in her own field. "He let me help with some of the treatments and I enjoyed the work and the patients so much that I went back to school." She says she has no regrets. She worked in direct patient care for two years after earning her bachelor of science degree in nursing and is now working toward her master's degree. She already has a position lined up as the nurse educator on her unit. While this speaks to the many opportunities that exist in nursing, it also further demonstrates healthcare's challenge. It is not enough just to attract bright, young, motivated people to nursing; they have to be given a reason to stay at the bedside. This means giving them the opportunity to exercise their critical thinking and decision-making skills at the point of care. From the management perspective, it means giving nurses the authority to make decisions about appropriate staffing, scheduling, and skill mix to meet the patients' needs and letting them choose which equipment is most important to purchase and when. And from physicians, it means allowing nurses to have more input into a patient's plan of care. Though many experienced nurses with excellent clinical skills stayed at the bedside in the past, it cannot be assumed it will happen in the future without substantial change.

But change doesn't have to be painful; nurse-physician relationships aren't beyond help and the benefits of change are far reaching. An interdisciplinary team approach to patient care, where the input of all team members (nurses, doctors, pharmacists, physical therapists, etc.) is valued, has the potential to positively affect nurse recruitment and retention. It can also increase patient safety and positively affect physician job satisfaction. The Institute of Medicine's 1999 report that raised the alarm about patient safety recommended interdisciplinary clinical practice as a means of decreasing medical errors. In 1998 the Pew Health Commission, a group funded by the Pew Charitable Trusts and administered by the Center for Health Professions at the University of California, issued a report outlining what they considered necessary changes to the healthcare system. The requirement for health professionals to learn to serve as part of interdisciplinary teams was one of them.[6] The study of magnet hospitals, those hospitals that created work environments that served to attract and retain nurses, demonstrated that patient safety was measurably enhanced in institutions promoting collaboration between members of the healthcare team.[7] Though not an element of the study, a secondary finding was that physicians reported that they enjoyed greater job satisfaction as well.

It all starts with the opportunity for increased communication. The University of California at Davis incorporated the inclusion of nurses on patient rounds with physicians, and both nurses and doctors were able to benefit from the shared knowledge.[8] While the doctors could teach about specific diagnoses, nurses often had information to share about prevention and treatment of hospital complications, such as skin breakdown. In a troubled Florida hospital, the hospital administration started by adopting a zero-tolerance policy for physician abuse of staff. In the emergency room, where patient satisfaction rates were low, besides shifting key personnel, the nurses began voting for a "Doctor of the Week." Though some thought it was frivolous, the result was that doctors began spending more time with the nurses as they vied for the title. Working relationships improved, patient satisfaction rates improved, and nursing turnover was reduced.[9]

The last decade hasn't been kind to physicians. Aside from the bewildering maze of managed-care plans and determining which plan will pay for what, Medicare has cut reimbursement to physicians in response to the Balanced Budget Act. Medical malpractice insurance premiums have soared to astronomical levels and the number of lawsuits filed is climbing. An obstetrics and gynecology physician in Las Vegas reported that his malpractice insurance rose from $33,000 per year in 2001 to $108,000 in 2002, forcing him to consider closing his practice. Between 1993 and 1999, the average medical malpractice award rose from $1.95 million to $3.5 million.[10]

Physicians are under siege. Asking for more concessions seems almost unkind. Yet if the nursing shortage is allowed to go unchecked it will impair the physicians' ability to practice. Already at some hospitals, procedures are limited and operating rooms stand empty due to a lack of skilled nurses to staff them. Working together to form a better partnership in care may be challenging, but the potential benefit for nurses, doctors, and patients has been demonstrated to outweigh the cost of the effort.

In the chapter that follows, the most important and most vulnerable member of the healthcare team will be considered. How has the nursing shortage impacted the patients who seek care?

NOTES

1. M. A. Manderino and N. Berkey, "Verbal Abuse of Staff Nurses by Physicians," *Journal of Professional Nursing* 13 (1997): 48–55

2. Alan H. Rosenstein, "Original Research: Nurse-Physician Relationships: Impact on Nurse Satisfaction and Retention," *American Journal of Nursing* 102, no. 6 (June 2002): 26–34.

3. Ibid.

4. Ibid.

5. Ibid.

6. "Recreating Health Professional Practice for a New Century," Pew Health Professions Commission [online], www.futurehealth.ucsf.edu [December 1998].

7. A. M. Rafferty, J. Ball, and L. H. Aiken, "Are Teamwork and Professional Autonomy Compatible, and Do They Result in Improved Hospital Care?" *Quality in Health Care* 10, suppl. 2 (2001): ii 33.

8. Josh Fischman, "Nursing Wounds: When Arrogant Docs Drive Nurses Away, Patients Suffer," *U.S. News & World Report*, June 17, 2002, pp. 54–55.

9. Ibid.

10. Mary Brophy Marcus, "Healthcare's 'Perfect Storm,'" *U.S. News & World Report*, July 1, 2002, p. 40.

CHAPTER SIX

And What about the Patient?

The amount of time a patient is allowed to remain in the hospital has decreased. Insurance payments have gone up and down (mostly down), new technology comes and goes, but one aspect of care has remained constant for nurses—their dedication to the patients and their desire to "make a difference" in patients' lives. When all else fails, it is concern for the patient that enables a nurse to work with the sights, sounds, and smells that repel others; to sacrifice time with a spouse or a family; to forgo meals; and to remain devoted to a job that is often physically and emotionally exhausting. Paperwork can rarely inspire that kind of dedication.

But what about the patients? Certainly there is no one on whom the current conditions have greater impact than the people whose injuries or illnesses force them to seek medical care. And for the vast majority of the American public, the changes in their healthcare came without warning. There were no consultants to walk them through the reasons for the decreased length of hospital stays, to explain why many surgeries had turned into one-day procedures, why the other patients in the hospital were so much sicker than they had been just a decade ago, or why the nurse disappeared for hours at a time. One day they (or a family member) were admitted to the hospital and discovered everything had changed since their last visit. So what does it feel like to be a patient under current conditions?

The following illustrates the healthcare experience of three patients admitted to the same nursing unit. Each offers a unique perspective.

Sue Crawford* was faced with the many issues of the "sandwich" generation, squeezed between the needs of adolescent children and aging parents. Her problem was compounded by location. She lived three states away from her parents. It worried her. When her father died of a sudden heart attack, Sue packed up her mother, Mildred Bedford, and moved her to a nearby retirement community where she could visit daily.

Initially, it seemed an ideal solution. It was a pleasant community, tree-lined and well landscaped, but the move created problems that Sue had never considered, including healthcare. She had presumed that her mother would be able to use the family physician that she herself had been seeing for years, but when she called, she was told that his practice had a full quota of Medicare recipients and couldn't accept any new ones. She telephoned seven different offices before finding a young physician, fresh out of residency, who would accept an additional Medicare patient.

There was more, of course. Her mother, who had always been so sociable, seemed disinterested in making new friends in the retirement community. Why bother, she would ask, when they were all old and were just going to die as her dear husband had. The young physician suggested an antidepressant, which Sue thought was a terrible idea, a glib and uncreative response to her mother's problem. She thought it was probably just because he didn't want to take the time to find any other solution. Her mother had surprised her by accepting the drug, however, and after a few weeks had seemed to act more like her old self. Then she had a stroke, and even though she was in a retirement community where there was some oversight, Mildred had lain on the ground for hours, unable to speak or move.

Finding a nursing home was a nightmare Sue hadn't prepared for, but her mother didn't get better. Her speech didn't come back and her mobility remained impaired. Her whole left side was lifeless and her face drooped on that side. After just a couple of days in the hospital, the doctor told Sue that her mother needed to be discharged, that it was

---

*Sue Crawford and the other characters in this chapter are fictitious, though the challenges they face are real.

time to find her some "extended-care facility" as he termed it, as if he had given up and lost interest in her.

The responsibility all fell on Sue. Though the facility that accepted her mother was the best place she could find, Sue suspected that her mother didn't get near the care she deserved, and with her inability to communicate she never could be sure. Sue had seen those television programs with the hidden cameras. She knew the kind of things people did to old people, to the vulnerable, especially women, and the thought of someone hurting her mother sickened her.

Then there was the awful day that she entered her mother's room and could see by the pink of her cheeks and her restlessness that she had a fever. Her lips were cracked and her skin dry as if she was dehydrated. Sue had had to threaten the nurse before she would come and then she had to wait hours for the young doctor to show up, but finally he'd admitted her mother to the hospital, where Sue thought that at least for a few days she would be safe.

Ron Paulson had a secret. He didn't have many opportunities for secrets anymore, now that he'd moved in with his daughter. She was good to him, there was no doubt, but it cost her having him there. He could see it; just the burden of another mouth to feed, the need for an extra bedroom when there was none to be had. The boys had to double up because he'd moved in.

Ron didn't have much feeling in his feet anymore. He'd had diabetes for years and hadn't given it much thought. He'd kept smoking though his doctor had advised him to stop and he ate pretty much what he wanted, figuring that was what insulin was for, to cover him when he ate a little too much candy or drank a couple of beers. He'd had to cut back on the smoking when he moved in with his daughter, though. She knew when he snuck one outside, even when he used breath mints. She said the smell stayed on his skin. She watched what he ate, too, but he could sneak what he wanted during the day when she was at work. She had too much to do, though, with her boys and work. And that was another reason he kept his secret: He didn't want his daughter to feel she had to take care of him.

It had started as just a little place, red and angry-looking, on his big toe. He hadn't paid much attention at first. At his age, red places were hardly worth noting. Red spots, brown spots, dry crusty spots—he had them all, but this one had turned into a fat blister and started to ooze. He tried to take care of it, emptying half a bottle of peroxide over top of the angry sore and watching it foam up a couple times a day. It didn't hurt, but it didn't get better and one evening when he took off his shoe, he thought he detected a bad odor. Then his daughter found the empty peroxide bottles in the trash and she came looking for him. She took one look at his foot and scolded him for keeping it a secret. Before he could catch his breath she had him in the doctor's office, which is how he ended up in the hospital on antibiotics, hoping he'd get to keep his foot.

Will Johnson didn't feel too bad about dying. Not that he liked the idea, but he was staring ninety-five in the face. He'd won so far as he could see. He'd outlived two wives and assorted other women friends. He'd done just about everything he'd imagined himself doing and then some. He'd gone to places he'd barely been able to pronounce and had made and lost more money than ten men put together. So dying was okay with him. At least most days it was okay. When he saw his grand-children and his great-grandchildren, he wasn't so sure. He wanted to see them grow. It was like leaving a movie before the ending. Still, death was wearing him down. He was getting tired of waiting. And the pain was starting to invade all his waking moments. The doctor had prom-ised him that she'd keep him comfortable and she'd tried to keep that promise with medication, but if Will took as much as he needed to be comfortable, he would fall asleep. And he didn't think he had enough time left to be wasting it on sleeping. It could be his last sunrise or last birdcall. He'd hate to miss it because of sleep. And medicated sleep wasn't even relaxing. It was fuzzy and murky, with crazy dull dreams of shadowy beings.

He'd been in and out of the hospital: short visits, mostly for chemotherapy or to receive blood transfusions to replace what the chemotherapy had taken from him. He'd told his doctor what he'd wanted: home time, freedom to be himself as long as possible, to drive, to go to the great-grandkids' ballgames, to stop at the diner for a cup of coffee and flirt with the waitresses. And he'd gotten just about all he'd asked for, but this morning the doctor had suggested it was time to take the keys away, to park his car, at least till his pain was under control. Will knew what that really meant. He didn't need it sugar-coated. He knew that giving up driving would be for the last time. Parking the car meant forever.

He'd thought he wanted to die in his own bed, but he'd seen the look on his son's face when he brought it up. He guessed what his son was thinking, that he would be alone when it happened, that no one would know if he slipped away. Dying alone was okay with him, but he didn't figure it was worth arguing about, so when his doctor suggested that he might be able to get the pain controlled better if he were in the hospital, he agreed to the admission. He took one last long look around his cozy house, at the picture of his first wife that he still kept by his bed, and then he took a final spin in his car, before the pain in his side made it hard even to breathe.

On the same day, all three of the above patients converged on Karen Hensley's unit: Will Johnson, Ron Paulson, and Mildred Bedford. Will Johnson was assigned to Emma, Ron Paulson to Lilly, and Mildred Bedford to Karen herself.

Mr. Johnson's needs were the least intense of the three. When he first entered the hospital, the nurses on Three West assessed his venous status and recommended to his physician that he have a PICC (a special type of long flexible IV access that is inserted in the inner forearm and carries fluid to a large vein near the heart) line inserted because it could remain in place for weeks without needing replacement. The physician agreed and also ordered a PCA (patient controlled analgesia) pump set up with morphine. A small amount of morphine ran continuously as a baseline rate to keep the edge off his pain and the PCA allowed Mr. Johnson to give himself small extra doses when the pain was especially great. Will liked the control it allowed him. When his grandchildren came by with the great-grandkids, he could just grit his teeth through the pain and manage to stay alert enough to enjoy the visit, but when they were gone, he didn't have to wait for a nurse to get some relief.

When he had learned that he was dying, he had contacted the local hospice organization that was dedicated to helping people with a limited lifespan to live out their time with dignity, emphasizing comfort measures and pain control rather than aggressive treatment. It made sense to him. He could see no advantage to more tests and chemotherapy when the cancer would inevitably take him. While he was at home, the hospice nurses had stopped in regularly. He had dreaded their visits initially, thinking that people who worked with the dying must be morbid, serious types with somber faces, but they had proved to be anything but somber. Though they asked the questions no one else seemed able to ask about how he envisioned death and encouraged him to communicate his desires about his funeral and disposition of his estate, they also joked and teased and listened to his stories. Most important to him, they seemed unoffended by the daily breakdown of his body, by the gas that escaped unheeded or his breath that tasted of his own decaying flesh. He could see the gauntness that came to his features reflected in the frightened eyes of his children and grandchildren. Some days they nearly winced to look at him, but it never seemed to bother the nurses. They understood his lack of appetite and his failing organs. And though they offered suggestions, they didn't press. They accepted his choices.

The hospice nurses didn't stop coming to see him when he went to the hospital. He could never say it, but it touched him that they didn't abandon him. The hospital nurses were good, and equally nonjudgmental, but they were hurried. He could almost hear the clock ticking as they cleaned his bed and helped him bathe, could feel the pull the world outside his room had on them, how they would stiffen at the crackle of the intercom over his bed. Sometimes they would leave suddenly, murmuring apologies, and then return later to finish their tasks. The weaker he got, the more efficient they seemed to get and they had eyes like hawks. They never missed a change in his breathing, a red spot on his skin, or his parched lips. Lotions were rubbed on his legs and feet, emollients on his lips, things he never would have allowed if he'd been able. But the closer to death he came, the less he cared to assert his boundaries, his independence. That their hands were soft and gentle was enough. The doctor came around with her chart and sat in the room sometimes. She asked about his pain, whether he was eating or drinking, but she acknowledged her role was diminishing. Mostly, she said, she counted on the nurses to tell her when they needed other medications or treatments ordered. She counted on them to keep Will comfortable.

Ron Paulson was worried. He could sense his control slipping as soon as he walked into the hospital. The nurse call bell they tied to his bed frame, the gown they wanted him to wear, the way they wanted him to be mindful of how he used his arm so that the IV site was protected, the tray of bland food that appeared—it all spoke to his loss of control. And the doctor had admonished him about not taking better care of his feet, about not being diligent enough with his inspections, as if he had any idea what it meant to try to inspect his feet when he was half blind and his back hurt too much to bend any closer. The doctor didn't say much either. He would come into the room and peer at Ron's foot and poke and mumble. After a couple of days, he sent in a surgeon, who took Ron down to the operating room and cut away at his toe, trying, he said, to get to the good tissue where the blood flow was still strong. The surgeon took him to the operating room two more times, but he didn't look very hopeful and one day he let the word "amputation" slip.

The very word distressed Ron. He had seen men with no legs riding around in wheelchairs, dependent on someone else to help them get to the chair and the bed, to move around the house. He couldn't afford that. There was no one to help him. His daughter would try her best and she'd push the grandsons to help, too, but it would be a terrible burden and he was already infringing far too much on their busy lives. So he kept the threat to himself and tried to look cheery when the family came around.

It was worse when Ron started thinking about the money. He'd already been in the hospital nine days, was getting two different antibiotics through the IV in his arm, had been to the operating room, and his doctor was talking about calling in a specialist on infectious disease. He could almost see the bills piling up. He bet every time one of those doctors entered his doorway, a new charge was added. It took his appetite away, all that worry. Forgetting to eat wasn't something he often did, but when his lunch tray came, he just pushed it aside. Then his IV infiltrated the soft tissue of his arm and Lilly came by and found it. She tried to restart it and he yelled at her for hurting him. Then things got dark.

The next thing Ron knew, someone had him by the shoulders and was shaking him. "Mr. Paulson, have you eaten since you took your insulin?" He tried to pull away. He raised his arm and swung drunkenly. "Leave me alone," he said, but the words were garbled.

Lilly was standing in front of him, pressing him to drink orange juice. "Mr. Paulson, you have to drink this now. You're having an insulin reaction. You have to drink this."

He tried to push her away, but Lilly stood firm. She said, "I want you to drink every drop. Now. And I'm not leaving till you do." He turned the cup and drank it down. "Another," she said just as firmly. He took the second cup in his hand and stared at it and then began drinking more slowly. Finally he sat back in his chair. His head was buzzing. "What happened?" he asked.

Lilly sat down on the edge of the bed. "You had an insulin reaction. You took your insulin this morning, remember? And you didn't eat. Do you have these often?"

Mr. Paulson leaned back in his chair. "Never. That's never happened to me before. I don't know what came over me. Did I hurt you? I wasn't trying to. Everything felt crazy."

Lilly said, "What do you know about your diabetes? If you take your insulin and then don't eat, this can happen. And do you carry something with you? Some little piece of candy, just in case?"

He shook his head.

"It's important for you to try to keep your blood sugar as even as possible. I'll order you a fresh lunch and you have to promise you'll eat it. How often do you check your own sugar?"

"The doctor does it when I go there."

Lilly stood up. "We're going to have to do some work this afternoon. I'll bring you a video and I want you to watch it and then we're going to talk about how your sugar affects your body and gives you infections like the one in your toe, but first I want you to eat a little something from this tray while I order you some hot soup."

"The doctor said he's got to take my foot," Ron blurted, relieved that he'd finally spoken his worry aloud.

Lilly frowned. "Are you sure? I think he's just talking about your toe right now. But if you don't take better care of yourself and check your sugar and eat well, it could be your foot next. We'll sit down together and I'll go over everything about your diabetes with you and what you need to do, but first I want you to eat and I need to check in on my other patients. Let's check your sugar now so we can get a better idea of what's going on. You gave us a good scare, you know."

He didn't say anything, but held out his hand to her so she could prick his finger and get a drop of blood for the glucometer. He spent the rest of the afternoon trying to think of a way to say thank you and finally picked up the phone to ask his daughter if it would be too inconvenient for her to make the nurses some of her famous cookies.

Sue Crawford was unimpressed with the care her mother, Mildred, received. She never saw a doctor the entire time her mother was in the hospital. When she mentioned it, the nurse just nodded and said that Mrs. Bedford's doctor normally conducted rounds early in the morning in order to get back to his office on time. Sue was incredulous that her mother could be in the hospital and not be seen by the doctor more often than that. The nurse said that she thought he sometimes came back after office hours, but she worked the dayshift so she couldn't be sure. It infuriated Sue that the nurse was so casual about it, as if it was acceptable, as if she should not have expected more.

Sue didn't think the nurses paid any attention to her mother either, since she couldn't talk. On the second day of her stay someone tied the call bell on the left side of the bed, on the same side as the arm that had been rendered useless by the stroke. When Sue told the nurse, the bell was moved and she was told that it had been left there by accident after the staff had turned Mrs. Bedford from her side, but she didn't believe it. Even if she had, it wasn't the kind of mistake they could afford to make. What if her mother needed them? Without a voice or a bell, and only the most cursory of checks on her, how would she get the assistance she needed?

In the evening when Sue went home, her mother was still restless, but when she came back in the morning and found her in urine-soaked sheets, she was nearly motionless and her breath sounded raspy. Her breakfast was stone cold on a tray that was far from her bed so that even if she'd had the energy to try to swallow a few mouthfuls, she wouldn't have been able to reach it.

After Sue complained, the nurse, Karen, came to her room and apologized for the oversight. She moved quickly to correct the problem, enlisting an aide to help turn Mrs. Bedford and scrub her clean. She ordered a new hot tray of food, though the patient hardly accepted a bite, and applied lotion to her dry skin and thin limbs. She even put special pads on her heels to protect the skin from breaking down, but Sue couldn't forgive her oversight. She knew her mother, her pride in being clean and tidy, and she was certain that with whatever awareness her mother possessed she was feeling the utter humiliation of the accident. Then Karen asked the question that upset her.

"Your mother doesn't have any antibiotics ordered that I noticed. Is she being treated for her pneumonia?"

"She has pneumonia? The doctor didn't say that. She didn't have it when she came here."

Karen pulled out her stethoscope and listened to Mildred's lungs. "She's breathing pretty rapidly and she's not exchanging much air. I can't say for sure, but I better call her doctor. Has your mother ever used oxygen before?"

Before Sue could answer, Karen left the room. She came back with tubing and a meter and put the oxygen tube up to her mother's face. "Mrs. Bedford, this will make you breathe a little easier. And I'm going to put the head of the bed up a little. That will help you, too. Do you think you could cough for me?"

Mrs. Bedford made a sound in her throat once and then again, but nothing that could be considered a cough. "This is hard for you, isn't it? Do you think you could try one more time? You've got some secretions building up in your lungs and you need to try to move them." She tried one more time and only hiccupped. Karen turned to Sue. "Was your mother able to get around with help before she came in?

Sue answered pointedly that her mother had been perfectly capable of using the toilet when someone bothered to help her get there, but the nurse didn't seem to even notice the ice in her tone. Karen voiced concern about Mildred's apparent deterioration from the independent woman Sue knew to a woman who was so weak that she could barely assist when they tried to turn her on her side.

Karen checked Mildred's blood pressure and pulse and raised the head of the bed a little more. She asked her to cough, but only a sound like a gurgle escaped.

"Can't you see how tired she is? She's been ill, you know. You do know that much, don't you?" Sue was starting to worry and she could barely keep civil. "When is the doctor coming?"

Karen clipped a device over the patient's finger and announced that her "sats were a little low" as if Sue should know what that meant. She went on to explain that the device read the level of oxygen in blood and that her mother's numbers were lower than that of people who don't have chronic respiratory diseases. She left the room saying she was going to call the doctor.

Soon after talking with the doctor, Karen came back with an IV bag of medicine and said that the doctor had ordered antibiotics. Then a respiratory therapist came in and thumped on Mrs. Bedford's back and made her inhale from a tube. He used the finger device again and said that her "sats looked a little better" and then he was gone. Mrs. Bedford's breathing did sound a little better, but Sue was still uneasy. She waited until dinnertime, but the doctor didn't come.

Will Johnson died that evening right after the shift changed, peacefully drifting off just as he'd wanted. His family couldn't say enough about the care he'd received. The doctor, the hospice volunteers and nurses, and the hospital nurses all seemed to blend for them into one seamless mix of skill and compassion, especially compassion. Once the diagnosis had been settled upon and it had been established that no known treatment could effect a cure, it was kindness and understanding that they had sought. According to the letter Mr. Johnson's son delivered to the hospital president, they had found it in abundance at his hospital. They never noticed the skill it took for the nurses to maintain his comfort as there was no obvious evidence in the form of high-tech equipment or complex technology. They saw the nurses touching and comforting him and were unaware of the assessment skills utilized in each touch or glance or of the critical thinking required to anticipate each physical change and act to prevent potential unpleasant symptoms. What they understood was that even though he died in a hospital, there was nothing cold or institutional about the way it happened. The patient and

his family were enveloped in caring and kindness. In the days that followed, the hospice nurses and chaplain stayed in touch. Some of the
family even took advantage of the bereavement support group. Though
they were acutely saddened by the absence of the man they loved, they
all remembered his death as a surprisingly uplifting event, a spiritual
passing of a man they didn't want to see suffer any longer.

Ron Paulson was discharged the following morning. His doctor told him
that he would need to continue his antibiotics, but that Medicare
wouldn't pay for him to be in the hospital for that. If it didn't get better,
he might have to have his toe removed, but first he would need to return
daily to the outpatient clinic for another five weeks of IV antibiotics. This
made Ron almost as distressed as thinking his whole foot would be
removed. He had no way to get to the hospital every day. Both his
daughter and son-in-law worked. But Emma and Lilly came to his rescue.
They contacted the hospital social worker, who arranged his rides.

Though the infection did not entirely resolve and he had to return
for surgery, only his toe was taken. He never regained the feeling in his
feet, but he did follow Lilly's advice. He started a walking program and
tried to eliminate the sweets from his diet. After a few months and a
weight loss of eighteen pounds, the doctor was able to decrease his
insulin dose and he found that he felt years younger. He gradually took
over the family cooking and meal planning and felt for the first time as
if he were really contributing to the household instead of taking from
it. He thought often of the nurses on Three West with real fondness—
especially Lilly, because she had saved his life.

Mildred Bedford was less fortunate. Later that evening, her doctor
phoned her daughter at home just as she was finishing the after-dinner
cleanup. Sue's boys had gone to their rooms to start their homework
and her husband had been dispatched to the convenience store for
milk, so she was alone in the kitchen.

"Mrs. Crawford?" he said. "This is Dr. Canville calling about your
mother, Mildred Bedford."

Sue immediately felt panicky. "Yes?" was all she could trust herself
to respond.

"I'm in the hospital seeing your mother and I'm afraid she is not doing very well. As you probably noticed this afternoon, her breathing is pretty weak and raspy. We sent her for a chest X ray and she definitely has pneumonia. And she's noticeably weaker. That's a bad sign. She's not coughing up the secretions that have settled in her lungs. She's not going to be able to continue breathing on her own for much longer."

Sue was stunned. "What are you saying?"

"We can move her to the Intensive Care Unit and put her on a ventilator. Certainly we can do that, but I can't guarantee it will change the outcome. She still may not live very long."

Sue felt as if she were suffocating. "Are you saying you expect her to die? I don't understand."

"Mrs. Crawford, your mother is eighty-three years old and has suffered a stroke. Now she has pneumonia and she just isn't strong enough to fight it. She either has to be put on a ventilator or we can make her comfortable. I had a pulmonologist see her this evening and he agreed, but we're getting to the time when a decision has to be made. The first time I saw your mother in my office, I asked about her wishes should she be in such a situation. I wrote in my notes that she didn't want any heroic measures, but she never signed anything that I know of. Did she ever talk to you about that?"

Sue didn't speak immediately. She was stunned by the finality in the doctor's voice. "Are you trying to say she's going to die tonight?"

"As I said, she's very weak. I don't know if she can make it through the night without assistance with her breathing. To help her, we'd have to put a tube down her throat and we'd probably have to sedate her some to keep from frightening her."

Sue was silent.

"Mrs. Crawford, do you want to take a few minutes and talk it over with your family? I can give you the number where I can be reached. I'll be in the hospital for at least another hour. I wouldn't wait too long, though."

It was a difficult decision, one that Sue didn't really agree with, but her husband thought that her mother wouldn't want to suffer, that it was better to allow her to go naturally. He pointed out that the doctor had discussed it with her and that she had indicated as much to him, but it wasn't so clear to Sue and she was the one who had to sit the night with her mother while she struggled for breath. The nurses tried to help. They gave Mrs. Bedford medication to ease her breathing and brought tea and a portable bed for Sue so she could rest, but she stayed awake until sunrise, until her mother had slipped away.

As the months passed, life returned to its routine for Sue Crawford. Her elder son acquired his learner's permit while the younger began to excel at soccer. For Sue, there remained a painful absence, though, a void her mother had once filled. She missed her mother's voice (the one she'd had before the stroke), her counsel, and her warm smile. And nothing could be settled. Her mother's personal effects were distributed, but her small estate was still paying bills. For months, it dragged on, bills arriving from the physicians, the nursing home, and the hospital, until one day the lawyer called and said that while outstanding bills remained, the estate was depleted. It was the final insult. Sue's story of the last days of her mother's life tumbled out, the dissatisfaction she felt about the care her mother had received and her suspicion that it was the inadequate attention from the nurses and doctors that ultimately caused her death. The lawyer listened quietly. When she was finished he told her that he could request copies of her mother's medical records if she wished. She agreed, but before hanging up she added that if they were to bring a suit against the hospital, she wanted to be certain that Karen Hensley and Dr. Canville were specifically named.

Whatever happens in healthcare, it is the patients who pay the highest price. The nurses feel overburdened, the physicians sense their autonomy slipping away, and executives wonder if they can continue to operate in the black, but it is the patients who fear for their own safety. In 1999 an Institute of Medicine report titled "To Err is Human" was released, and its conclusion received much notice in the popular press. It estimated that between forty-four thousand and ninety-eight thousand Americans died annually from medical errors, more than from automobile accidents.[1] Though many physician and nursing groups questioned the results of the study, it was enough to send chills down the spines of Americans faced with imminent hospitalization. Would their health be more imperiled by the hospitalization than their disease?

Some might think so. A study published in the *Archives of Internal Medicine* in September 2002 and covered in the *Philadelphia Daily News* reported that hospitals average more than forty potentially harmful errors each day,[2] frequently involving the administration of medication. According to the researchers, errors occurred in nearly one of five doses of medication. Usually involving errors of omission (not giving the medication at all) or giving the medication at the wrong time, they were related specifically to nurses since the errors occurred during actual administration of the drugs and not during their preparation or ordering.[3] In a survey released by the Harvard School of Public Health and the Kaiser Family Foundation, 42 percent of the public and more than a third of doctors reported that they or a family member had experienced a medical error. Both groups cited overworked, fatigued health-care workers as a major factor in the error.[4]

In 2002 two studies were released that documented the impact of nurse staffing on the health status of the hospitalized patient. A University of Pennsylvania study concluded that the nurse-to-patient ratio had a significant effect on patient health. For every extra patient assigned to a registered nurse over the baseline, the patients in her care were at a 7 percent greater risk of death within thirty days of admission.[5] So if she were assigned two extra patients, the risk grew to 14 percent. Though for most patients, the impact of greater patient-to-nurse ratios means inconvenience—longer waiting times for nurses to reply to call bells for pain medicine or bathroom assistance—the results can be devastating. At the very least, the release of the study increases patient anxiety. A cartoon in the *Richmond Times-Dispatch* by Stahler may summarize the uneasy feelings in America. A nurse with a chart is standing before a gravestone. She addresses it saying, "Sorry I couldn't get here sooner . . . nurse shortage, you know."

Mr. Johnson, Mrs. Bedford, and Mr. Paulson had hospital admissions that were impacted by a number of factors, including the number of nurses on the unit. A closer analysis reveals how increased nurse staffing might or might not have helped in each situation.

Mr. Johnson felt the lack of staffing the least. Aside from his IV and PCA pump for pain, he had no unusual medications, did not require diagnostic procedures or tests, and had an attentive family with round-the-clock visits. Since he had signed on with hospice, he had already agreed that no aggressive curative treatments would be performed, only comfort measures, so there was no chemotherapy to administer. The hospice nurses who had been following him at home still made visits and had taken the time before his admission to explain some of what might happen during the dying process, so there was little critical patient instruction required of the hospital nurses. Mr. Johnson's oncologist was well known to the nursing staff and was easily accessible for consultations about increasing pain medications or adding medications that would decrease his secretions if needed for easier breathing. Everyone involved, including nurses, doctors, the patient, and his family, was clear about what to expect. Though the end result was Will's death, a sad experience for everyone involved, his hospital stay was not adversely affected by the shortage of nurses.

There were no definitive errors involved in Mr. Paulson's admission and he was ultimately satisfied with the outcome. There was no indication that medication doses were omitted or that he felt he had not been given adequate attention. After all, Lilly did save his life, and stayed with him through a very frightening event. She spent the rest of the afternoon explaining his diabetes to him as well, even staying beyond her shift. By the time she was done, she had asked the doctor to prescribe a glucometer for him, had talked to his daughter about his diabetes, and had convinced Ron never to skip a meal and to carry an emergency sugar source in case he had too much insulin. From his point of view, his hospitalization had a good outcome.

But what would the nurses say? From their perspective, it was his ninth day in the hospital and still the nurses were unaware that he had very little real knowledge of his disease. From the nurses' point of view, they shouldn't have had to save him from his insulin reaction, but rather could have prevented the problem if they had had the time to assess his knowledge and intervene earlier. Even if his lack of information hadn't been discovered, a nurse who had had time to check on him more regularly would have seen the uneaten tray of food and recognized impending trouble. Though Lilly did ultimately teach him about his diabetes, she had to stay for two hours of overtime to fit it in. So overall, he did not directly suffer injury as a result of an overworked nursing staff, but that was due to luck.

Mrs. Bedford's case is more difficult. She entered the hospital from the nursing home with a fever of unknown origin. The fever may have been an indication of an infection brewing or may have created the environment that was a perfect breeding ground for the bacteria that caused the pneumonia. Her stroke may have impaired her swallowing and left her vulnerable to aspiration pneumonia (a lung infection caused when food particles accidentally enter the airway). It's impossible to tell from the scenario presented at exactly what point that would have happened, but she was admitted without active pneumonia and ultimately died in the hospital of its complications. Whether the source of her lung infection was a bug acquired in the nursing home or in the hospital, more staffing and therefore more frequent assessments could certainly have facilitated an earlier intervention and possibly saved her life. Even if a cure was not the intended outcome, that is, if Mrs. Bedford, like Mr. Johnson, was going to require only comfort care to ease her into death, an inadequate amount of care was given. Leaving the call bell out of reach of a person who lacks speech or mobility is a recipe for disaster, and assistance with toileting should never be overlooked but can happen easily when nurses are assigned too many patients.

Another important issue is Sue Crawford's expectations. Mrs. Bedford was eighty-three years old, had recently lost her husband, had been depressed, and had lost her speech and mobility due to the stroke. Her long-term prognosis was poor and very likely apparent to her doctor, but not to Sue Crawford, her daughter. While perhaps one might ask what outcome Sue was realistically expecting for her mother—certainly she was not going to regain the life she had before the stroke—the minimal communication between the doctor and the patient's family certainly contributed to Sue's lack of understanding. Managing the health expectations of patients and their families is especially important as medicine becomes more complex and resuscitation efforts and well-publicized medical advances mislead the public into believing a cure is always possible. Then when an inevitable death occurs, the family may feel betrayed by the healthcare system, a situation that takes on even more importance at a time when lawsuits are not uncommon. In the case of Mrs. Crawford, if the nurses had had the time to spend with her and assess her understanding of her mother's condition, they could have alerted the doctor. Ultimately for Mrs. Bedford and her daughter, too many patients per nurse had a decidedly detrimental effect.

To this point, it has been established that nurses are dissatisfied with their working conditions, some are leaving the profession, and fewer new nurses are entering the profession to replace those who leave. In addition, the resulting nursing shortage is likely to worsen as the health needs of baby boomers increase. The vignettes offered in this chapter illustrate what fewer nurses could actually mean in terms of patient care. If there are not enough nurses, care will certainly be compromised and it is the individual patients who will pay the greatest price. That makes the next question all the more important: How will the trend be reversed before it reaches even more critical proportions?

NOTES

1. "Medical Errors: The Scope of the Problem," Agency for Healthcare Research and Quality [online], www.ahcpr.gov/qual/errback.htm [February 2000].

2. Associated Press, "Study: Hospitals Make 40 Drug Goofs a Day," *Philadelphia Daily News*, September 9, 2002, p. 31.

3. Ibid.

4. "Harvard University Study Identifies Inadequate Nurse Staffing as a Major Factor in Medical Errors," American Nurses Association [online], http://nursingworld.org/pressrel [December 16, 2002].

5. "Busier Nurses, Riskier Hospitals?" CBSNews [online], www.cbsnews.com/stories/2002/10/22/health [October 22, 2002].

CHAPTER SEVEN
Enhancing the Workplace
HOW HOSPITALS RETAIN NURSES

I t would be easy to get stuck in the process of assigning blame for the apparent shortage of nurses, but discovering how things got off track is useful only if it offers a roadmap to the preferred destination. In other words, Where do we go from here?

Hospitals are facing the most pressure when it comes to a scarcity of nurses. In a 2001 survey, 89 percent of hospitals reported a shortage of registered nurses. Though other shortages have come and gone, this one has the potential to last into the foreseeable future. Often in the past, nursing shortages were related to boom economies that allowed some full-time nurses to drop to part-time status or to stay home altogether. A downturn in the economy or a large enough increase in wages could often entice them out of their temporary retirement, but this time the shortage is not based merely on economic factors that can be overcome by big sign-on bonuses. Nurses who are working in hospitals express deep dissatisfaction and they are no longer held captive by a lack of other opportunities. Women who traditionally staffed nursing units are finding that gender is no longer a career barrier in almost any sector of employment.

Nursing schools have seen a general decline in enrollment since 1995. In 2001 bachelor's degree programs saw an increase in enrollment for the first time in six years, but associate's degree enrollments continued to slide.[1] In past years, the trend would not have been alarming, but the baby boomers—the large bulge of post–World War II babies—are aging and their healthcare needs are increasing. In 2001 consumer spending on healthcare increased 8.7 percent, representing the largest increase in a decade and reflecting greater use of hospitals and prescription drugs.[2] The boomers did not produce children in the same record numbers as their parents, however, and the generation coming up is smaller in number and less inclined to enter fields that have been traditionally female. This is demonstrated by the average age of the nurse, which reached forty-seven in 2000.[3] Only 9 percent of nurses are currently under thirty, the group that is the most likely to staff hospitals.[4]

So what is a hospital to do? As any commodity becomes scarce, the price goes up. This is true whether we are speaking of widgets or of a desired skill. Nurses whose wages have been stagnant for a decade and whose roles have been redefined at the whim of cost-cutting consultants and HMOs are now awakening to a new sense of power. The hospitals that previously laid nurses off and forced those who remained to work overtime to compensate will likely have to pay for their folly. They can expect to enter bidding wars for nurses and may have to pay extra-large "memory" bonuses just to help hires forget their recent past. For the majority of institutions that simply did not recognize the impact of increased acuity on the nursing staff and have scurried to compensate, there is another, less expensive alternative—retaining the workforce they have.

The Art of Retention and Recovery

The findings of Julie Sochalski, associate professor at the University of Pennsylvania, suggest that methods for retention and for recovering already trained nurses who have left nursing may be at least as important and cost effective as strategies for recruiting new nurses.[5] In the United States in 2000, there were an estimated 2.7 million licensed registered nurses. Eighty-two percent were employed as nurses (28 percent of those were working part-time).[6] This means that 18 percent—nearly half a million RNs—who are already trained and licensed constitute a resource waiting to be tapped. By creating an inviting work environment, hospitals could potentially lure these nurses back into the workforce.

To get them back, however, there needs to be an understanding of why they left. Some half million nurses have simply retired but kept their licenses active. Of the others, nearly 81,000 left their jobs to stay home with young children. Another 40,000 moved into new careers; the reasons they most often cited for doing so included better wages, better hours, and more rewarding work.[7] It is possible then that 120,000 RNs could be enticed back to hospitals by providing childcare, flexible hours, increased pay, and more opportunity for meaningful promotion that would recognize their expertise without taking them from the bedside.[8] That doesn't count the 28 percent of nurses working part-time who could make a significant impact if they could be enticed to increase their hours.

To get a better sense of why strategies to retain nurses are so essential, one has only to compare nurse job satisfaction with the level of satisfaction enjoyed in other segments of the workforce. In a survey of RNs in 2000, 69.5 percent reported being at least moderately satisfied with their jobs,[9] whereas a general survey of American workers conducted between 1988 and 1998 showed that 86 percent of general workers and 88 percent of professional workers reported being satisfied with their work.[10] The reasons cited by the nurses for their lack of enthusiasm were not related to patient care; in fact, the more time spent in patient care, the more satisfaction staff nurses reported. Instead, their unhappiness was related to their feeling of having little if any control over many aspects of their work. This carries over to new nurses as well, particularly among men who have gone into nursing. The percentage of men who drop out of nursing within four years of graduating rose from 2 percent in 1992 to 7.5 percent in 2000. In the same time period, women dropout rates rose from 2.7 percent to more than 4 percent.[11] As reported earlier, 23 percent of RNs indicated that they actively discouraged others from entering the nursing profession. It is not unlikely that a direct relationship exists between that negative recommendation and the reason new nurses exit the profession. New recruits do not last in an environment where their experienced coworkers (and potential mentors) are cynical and unhappy. Therefore, spending money on recruitment efforts is useless unless the focus first shifts to one devoted to retaining the nurses we have.

One workplace issue for nurses is the lack of safety equipment, for both patient and nurse safety. To enhance patient safety, computer systems that allow for direct order entry by physicians can slash medication errors and reduce the time spent calling physicians to double-check handwriting, while the bar coding of medications reduces errors that occur at the point of administration. Systems that allow for bedside documentation leave nurses with more time to spend with the patients. Nurses also fear for their own safety on the job and desire protection from inadvertent needlesticks as well as crippling back injuries. Many institutions have adopted safe needle devices (surveyed nurses reported 82 percent have safe needle devices available to them),[12] but according to the Centers for Disease Control and Prevention, the nation's obesity rate climbed to nearly 21 percent in 2002, a full percentage point higher than the previous year.[13] Since obesity is a major risk factor for many chronic diseases, a disproportionate number of obese people are likely to seek care, increasing nurses' risk for back injury unless proper lifting equipment and time to learn to use it are available. In an online survey, 54 percent of the nurses responded that patient lifting and transfer devices were not readily available for use and 60 percent listed a disabling back injury as one of their greatest safety concerns.[14] Although certified nurse's assistants may be available to help, they also are subject to injury in such a physical job.

COMPETITIVE WAGES

It is important to note that although wages for nurses were increased following the last shortage in the 1980s, between 1992 and 2000 wages barely moved when adjusted for inflation. In fact, the earning power of nurses did not increase at all.[15] While money is not the strongest draw for nurses, the implication of appreciation and value that is attached to wages is. Even in times of cost containment, there has to be some salary recognition for nurses to compete with other areas of employment.

Nurses are drawn to their field by the ability to "make a difference." Because of that intrinsic quality—the same that is attached to other types of service employment, such as teaching and social work— employers have been allowed to take their loyalty for granted, aware that it wasn't merely the benefits they offered that kept nurses dedicated to their work. But while that may have been true in the past, the climate has changed.

CREATING A MEANINGFUL WORKPLACE

To keep skilled nurses and use their satisfaction as a recruitment tool to attract others, healthcare leaders must "create work environments that are meaningful to their employees."[16] The Gallup organization, which has interviewed more than a million employees in the last twenty-five years, discovered twelve questions that they felt were most likely to measure the core elements needed in the workplace to attract and retain the most talented employees:

1. Do I know what is expected of me at work?
2. Do I have the materials and equipment I need to do my work right?
3. At work, do I have the opportunity to do what I do best every day?
4. In the last seven days, have I received recognition or praise for doing good work?
5. Does my supervisor, or someone at work, seem to care about me as a person?
6. Is there someone at work who encourages my development?
7. At work, do my opinions seem to count?
8. Does the mission/purpose of my company make me feel my job is important?
9. Are my coworkers committed to doing quality work?
10. Do I have a best friend at work?
11. In the last six months, has someone at work talked to me about my progress?

12. This last year, have I had opportunities at work to learn and grow?[17]

When distributed to various groups of employees, questions that are answered five on a one-to-five scale where five indicates "strongly agree" correlate to the "strength of the workplace in productivity, profitability, retention, and customer satisfaction."[18]

Comparing this list to the responses given on the nursing surveys gives a quick indication of where the problems lie. Nurses felt their opinions were unheard, that their work went unnoticed, that there were too many barriers that impeded them from doing their best, that they didn't always have the equipment needed, and that their hospital's mission had more to do with money than quality care. There is no assertion that the nurses' perception represents the real truth of their employer's intentions, but when considering retention of employees, their perception is all that matters.

FOCUS ON MANAGEMENT

Effective management is the key. According to the authors of *First, Break All the Rules*, the most important indicator of employee turnover is the employee's immediate manager.[19] Management skills may be an area where hospitals can benefit from development. Nurse managers, the direct supervisors of many staff nurses, are often nurses whose excellent clinical skills earned them a promotion. They may have received very little management training, however, and may be unskilled in both supervision and finance. That may be further complicated by another, more subtle factor: that when given power, nurses may be unskilled in sharing power with their coworkers.[20] Of equal importance is the fact that senior management staff are often totally lacking in clinical experience. In surveys, nurses indicated that they felt distanced from their nonclinical leaders, who were making decisions based on numbers with little idea of what work the nurses performed or how their management decisions affected the work. Matthew J. Lambert III, MD, MBA, FACHE (Fellow of the American College of Healthcare Executives), senior vice president for clinical operations of a midwestern hospital, is uniquely qualified to comment. As a surgeon who became a hospital executive, he has had the opportunity to experience both years of working side by side with nurses and acting as a member of senior management. He agrees with the nurses that the lack of clinical background at the CEO/COO level has been a "contributing factor in the erosion of trust within the nursing workforce . . . reflected in some of the arbitrary downsizing, tinkering with skill mix, and reengineering" of the 1990s. He says that in a former position, he was forced to counter "a consultant's recommendation that nurses be required to clean rooms so that the environmental services staff could be reduced." Executives who had any real understanding of the nurse's role in complex patient care would not even have entertained such a suggestion.

Hospital management teams will certainly be facing some significant challenges in the upcoming decade, and managers on all levels will require support. The next generation of leaders will need the following qualities as suggested by VHA, Inc. (a nationwide network of community-owned healthcare systems): understanding of customer needs and expectations, ability to manage quality and financial data, human resource skills, strategic visioning and planning, as well as marketing and continuous quality improvement skills.[21] For those managers who don't have the skills, facilities will need to help develop them with real training programs that bring in outside instructors for concentrated periods and follow up with regular refresher courses. It will be costly, but the capital expended is likely to pay off in big rewards if staff turnover is positively affected.

The hospitals most likely to retain their workforce in the future will also encourage their executive staff to spend time with their clinical staff for a "gut-level" understanding of the work required. Several VHA hospitals have begun programs that encourage greater leadership visibility among their employees, including periodic question-and-answer sessions for staff with senior management. Orlando Regional Healthcare has "introduced 'walk in my shoes' events where executives fulfill staff roles for a day."[22] Because of the nature of nursing, the importance of what they do can be misunderstood without observation. Until recent nursing research attached real numbers to the complications prevented, the surveillance required by nurses to ensure that patients didn't suffer postoperative complications or that a quick intervention was begun if they did has been largely invisible. Senior management staff's willingness to share in the actual experience can not only enhance their understanding but positively affect the nurses' perception of their investment in quality. Consider the alternative.

THE COST OF RN TURNOVER

The real-dollar cost of turnover for any personnel is high; for highly skilled workers, it is even higher. Just considering replacement costs in terms of recruitment, advertising, interviewing, orientation of a new employee, moving expenses, and so on, it is estimated that the cost of replacement of an RN is between 80 and 100 percent of his first year's salary. The average annual salary of an RN in 2001 was $46,000. At 87 percent, that is $40,000 per RN.[23] If a hospital employs five hundred RNs and has a 15 percent turnover rate, that translates to a cost of $3 million a year for replacing the nurses who left. Using the entire VHA hospital system employing 275,000 RNs as a larger example, at a 15 percent turnover rate the cost would equal $1.6 billion per year,[24] added to the already staggering annual cost of healthcare. And there are other associated costs. According to the VHA, workforce shortages cause hospitals to reduce available beds, cancel or delay surgeries, and experience severe overcrowding in their emergency rooms. Obviously, at the same time, high turnover and vacancies in nursing positions also impact the quality of services provided and patient satisfaction. In a VHA, Inc. study, facilities with a nurse turnover rate of between 22 percent and 44 percent had a higher mortality and longer average length of hospital stay than facilities with a lower nurse turnover. Those facilities with the higher turnover rate also saw a *36 percent increase in cost per patient discharge.*[25] In other words, it costs the high-turnover hospitals 36 percent more to give care to each patient than a hospital with lower nurse turnover. Remembering the Medicare DRG system where a hospital is paid a set amount per diagnosis regardless of cost, that extra cost has to be absorbed by the hospital. Hospitals with high turnover and vacancies also risk losing their other employees by requiring extra work of them, which in turn leads to more vacancies, creating a downward trend that could spiral.

THE BIDDING WARS

As the nursing shortage continues and populations shift, the nurses and the nursing schools are not always at the point of need. In desperate attempts to bolster their workforce, hospitals are using job fairs, advertisements, and even billboards to get their message out—they need nurses and they are willing to pay. And do they pay! Signing bonuses are increasingly popular tools, sometimes in dramatic figures, especially for the hard-to-recruit specialty areas such as intensive care and the operating room where experience is imperative. One Ohio hospital began offering $30,000 bonuses payable over three years, in April 2002, for nurses with specialized skills.[26] Others are paying varying amounts from a few thousand to $10,000. In one Florida hospital, the incentive isn't in the form of a signing bonus, but a down payment for a house. Still others offer thousands of dollars in the form of continuing education incentives for nurses wishing to earn more-advanced degrees. Though many hospitals cite their programs as being successful, even recruiting from several states away, it remains to be seen what the long-term effect will be. People who will be tempted by a signing bonus can just as likely be tempted by another when their tenure is over.

HEALTHCARE FOR THE AGING

In states that have created a business out of attracting retirees to the sunshine, an unforeseen crisis is looming. The same people who were lured to the sunshine by the ability to enjoy the benefits of outdoor living may find that paradise has its limits. Nationwide, about 12 percent of the population is over sixty-five. In at least five Florida counties that number hovers around 30 percent.[27] Considering that 77 percent of all cancers occur after age fifty-five, the implications for healthcare needs are obvious, but add to that the increasing rates of arthritis, joint replacements, and heart disease and the number grows more alarming. Will there be enough nurses in the right distributions? According to the National Center of Workforce Analysis report of July 2002, Florida is not yet in trouble, but in Arizona, another popular retirement state, nursing vacancy rates are above 15 percent.[28]

MAGNET HOSPITALS

One program that hospitals are turning to as a model for organizational structure is the magnet hospital program. In a traditional hospital environment, all major decisions about a nurse's work environment, from scheduling to budgeting to care guidelines, are determined by management, leaving the nurse at the bedside with little control over his practice. A magnet hospital is one in which there exists a participative management style that is characterized by involvement of staff at all levels. Communication is practiced in all directions and departments are decentralized so that nurses have a strong sense of control over their immediate environment and their daily work design. Autonomy is encouraged and supported and the staff nurses are accountable for their work practice design. Quality is a way of life and always focused on continuous improvement. Education is valued on all levels. Nurses are expected to seek continuing education and share their knowledge with less-experienced nurses and with their patients. And their relationship with physicians is collegial, demonstrating mutual respect for one another's role in quality patient care. The description almost sounds too good to be true, but magnet hospitals are getting a lot of attention. A study conducted by Linda Aiken, PhD, RN, who directs the Center for Health Outcomes and Policy Research at the University of Pennsylvania in Philadelphia, demonstrated that compared to nonmagnet hospitals, magnet hospitals have some very desirable outcomes. These include Medicare patient mortality rates by 4.6 percent, a 60 percent higher likelihood of AIDS patients leaving the hospital alive, fewer potentially costly and deadly needlestick injuries suffered by nurses, higher patient satisfaction scores, belief by the nurses that the care the patients received was better than at other facilities, and higher nurse retention rates.[29] The American Nurses Certification Center certifies hospitals for magnet recognition after hospitals complete a comprehensive application and undergo a visit by surveyors. The rewards are high. As nurses hear more about the magnet hospitals, they are drawn to them as employers of choice. And the designation attracts patients as well. As of this writing, fifty-eight of the nearly nine thousand hospitals in the country are designated as magnet hospitals. Obviously, achieving magnet status isn't simply a matter of offering words of support. Everyone from the CEO to the CNA has to understand its implications. First and foremost, the power shifts to the point of care. And senior management needs to decide ahead of time how it will respond when it disagrees with a decision made by the staff nurses. If senior management overrules a decision, it has to be prepared to defend its position or risk killing the program.

EDUCATION INCENTIVES

For hospitals that are successful in changing the workplace either by achieving magnet status or by simply emulating some of the magnet program's qualities, the recruitment effort toward developing new talent will be much easier. A happy workforce is the best recruitment tool. One retention effort that many hospitals are offering, incentives for associate's degree and diploma nurses to return to school and earn their bachelor's degrees, may have an unexpected payoff. In a comparison of nurses in 2000, those with a bachelor of science degree in nursing as opposed to an associate's degree averaged an additional 2.2 years of work experience. The difference is even greater for nurses who began work with an AD and then returned to school to earn their BSN after. Those BSN nurses averaged 4.5 years of work experience more than those with a terminal AD.[30] With these statistics in mind and with the emphasis on education that is encouraged in a magnet facility, hospitals may benefit from giving financial incentives to their own employees before offering the same funding to recruits. And with the online programs now available the disruption to schedules may be minimal.

GIVING NURSES A VOICE

One recruitment and retention tool suggested by Matthew J. Lambert III is that hospitals invite more nurses to sit on their boards. "Why should such membership be limited to community members and physicians? Nurses need to be as much a part of decision making in the hospital environment as administrators and physicians. As the largest percentage of the workforce, they hold the key to both patient satisfaction and clinical quality." Certainly in hospitals that are striving toward the qualities of a magnet facility, representation of nurses on the governing boards sends a strong message to nurses about their value.

ATTRACTING THE YOUTH

Even with the lowest turnover rates, it is clear that nurses as well as other key hospital staff will need to be recruited in order to replace the staff that will be reaching retirement. Recruitment efforts can range from the tried-and-true to the truly creative. Keeping in the mind the characteristics of the generations following the baby boomers, it is unlikely that long-term commitment will be garnered just with words. They will need to believe in the mission of the institution and feel that their contributions are recognized. The self-sacrificing nurse is an outdated image that the younger nurses will not mold themselves into. They will, however, respond to programs that signal the possibility for maintaining balance in their lives. Flexible scheduling is an obvious choice, but other, more creative programs that some hospitals are promoting are free massage therapy or exercise programs for the staff, along with yoga classes or other forms of stress reduction. On the most emotionally taxing units, support groups offer nurses an opportunity to share their feelings and avoid the sense of being overwhelmed that can lead to burnout. A hospital in Asheville, North Carolina, has even partnered with the mortgage lender Fannie Mae to develop a home ownership program for employees.[31] The loyalty potential in that type of program can last a lifetime.

RECRUITING THE UNDERREPRESENTED

During recruitment efforts, hospitals need to look to the underrepresented in the field of nursing: men and minorities. Of the total number of nurses in America in the year 2000, 95 percent were women and 87 percent were white. Both for the richness that diversity brings to any workforce and to fairly mirror the diversity of the population, hospitals should be concentrating their efforts on the underrepresented. Some hospital groups are teaming together to bring their message of opportunity to schools, even as young as the elementary level. Yet another movement has been to actively recruit in other countries.

RECRUITING OUTSIDE OUR BORDERS

According to a *USA Today* story that appeared in September 2002, some twenty-three thousand foreigners took the nursing licensing exam in the United States last year. More than half came from the Philippines.[32] The nurse employment firms speak of recruiting outside our borders as one viable solution to the shortage, as well as an opportunity to raise the standard of living for some women. Others disagree just as strongly, pointing out that there are real problems in nursing that need to be fixed, not just worked around by recruiting nurses who will accept the current conditions because they are better than the conditions they are leaving behind. Others see it as an ethical issue. By hiring trained nurses from other countries, the problem is simply being transferred from America to their countries of origin. South Africa is one country from which nurses are being heavily recruited, in part because in South Africa, as in the Philippines, many recruits already speak English. Yet in South Africa, the citizens are contending with their own health issue, the AIDS crisis. Is this a country Americans should be taking nurses from, a country desperate for good healthcare personnel? It is a trend that bears notice.

A BRIGHTER FUTURE

Though much remains to be done and many challenges lie ahead as the healthcare system is pressed to care for increasing numbers of aging citizens, there are indications that the leadership is moving in the right direction. Of the fifty-eight facilities awarded magnet recognition by the American Nurses Credentialing Center since the program began, twenty were awarded in 2002 alone,[33] proving that interest is on the rise and that some institutions are beginning to demonstrate their appreciation for their nurses in tangible ways. And it may be having some real effects. In the 2000 survey of nurses, the new entrants into the workforce were the most satisfied. Compared to the 69.5 percent of the nurses overall indicating moderate satisfaction with their jobs, the new entrants posted a 75 percent satisfaction level.[34] Those levels certainly could sink over time, but if changes in practice are undertaken quickly, their satisfaction may soar because they won't have the negative conditions of the past to taint their current outlook.

Even though the hospitals, as employers, are perceived as holding all the power, it is apparent that the balance is shifting. As hospitals move to a new model of care, nurses will bear an increasing responsibility for building a bright future for the profession, as will be discussed in the next chapter.

NOTES

1. Julie Sochalski, "Nursing Shortage Redux: Turning the Corner on an Enduring Problem," *Health Affairs* 21, no. 5 (2002): 157–63.

2. Robert Pear, "Spending on Health Care Increased Sharply in 2001," *New York Times* [online], www.nytimes.com/2003/01/08/health/08HEAL.html [January 8, 2003].

3. AHA Commission on Workforce for Hospitals and Health Systems, *In Our Hands: How Hospital Leaders Can Build a Thriving Workforce*, April 2002.

4. Sochalski, "Nursing Shortage Redux," p. 157.

5. Ibid., pp. 157–63.

6. Robert Steinbrook, "Nursing in the Crossfire," *New England Journal of Medicine* 346, no. 22 (May 30, 2002): 1757.

7. Sochalski, "Nursing Shortage Redux,"

8. Ibid.

9. Ibid.

10. Ibid.

11. Ibid.

12. "Health & Safety Survey," *Nursing World* [online], http://nursing-world.org/surveys/hssurvey.pdf [September 2001].

13. "Obesity, Diabetes on Rise in U.S.," CBSNews [online], www.cbsnews.com/stories/2002/12/31/health [December 31, 2002].

14. "Health & Safety Survey."

15. Ibid.

16. Lilliee Gelinas and Chuck Bohlen, *Tomorrow's Work Force: A Strategic Approach*, VHA Research Series, 2002.

17. Marcus Buckingham and Curt Coffman, *First, Break All the Rules* (New York: Simon & Schuster, 1999), p. 28.

18. Ibid., p. 32

19. Ibid., p. 33.

20. Tim Porter-O'Grady, "Is Shared Governance Still Relevant?" *JONA* 31, no. 10 (October 2001): 468.

21. Gelinas and Bohlen, *Tomorrow's Workforce*, p. 16.

22. Ibid., p. 18.

23. Roger Herman, Tom Olivo, and Joyce Gioia, *Impending Crisis: Too Many Jobs, Too Few People* (Winchester, Va.: Oakhill Press, 2003), p. 166.

24. Ibid.

25. Ibid., p. 165.

26. Michael Janofsky, "Shortage of Nurses Spurs Bidding War in Hospital Industry," *New York Times*, May 28, 2002. Available [online], www.pef.org/nurses/shortage_of_nurses_spurs_bidding_war. htm [October 13, 2003].

27. Fred Brock, "That Long Shadow in the Sunshine State," *New York Times* [online], www.nytimes.com/2002/03/03/business/yourmoney/03SENI.html [March 3, 2002].

28. "Projected Supply, Demand, and Shortages of Registered Nurses: 2000–2020," U.S. Dept. of Health and Human Services [online], http://bhpr.hrsa.gov/healthworkforce/rnproject/report.htm [July 2002].

29. AHA Commission on Workforce, *In Our Hands*, p. 18.

30. Sochalski, "Nursing Shortage Redux," p. 162.

31. Gelinas and Bohlen, *Tomorrow's Workforce*, p. 24

32. Steve Friess, "Nursing Crisis at Crossroads: Foreign Hires Aren't Cure-alls for U.S. Ills, " *USA Today*. Available [online], www.stevefriess.com/archive/usatoday/nuring.htm [September 17, 2002].

33. Kay Bensing, "Lights on the Horizon," *Advance for Nurses* 4, no. 25 (December 2002): 43.

34. Sochalski, "Nursing Shortage Redux," p. 161.

CHAPTER EIGHT

Nurses

CREATING SOLUTIONS

Amiddle-aged woman was admitted from Emergency to a medical-surgical unit. She appeared dazed and picked absently at the tape that held the IV in her arm as she was transported by stretcher to her room. Jill Rhodes, the RN assigned to her room, entered behind the stretcher. "Hey, who is this? I didn't get report of anyone coming."

The orderly set the brake. "This is Mrs. Garrison. Can you help me move her and then I'll give you the report."

They tucked Mrs. Garrison into bed, her dress and stockings still in place. She didn't say anything. Her hair was disheveled, her clothes in disarray, and spittle was collecting in the corners of her mouth. She looked from one to the other and back again with lips pursed, but no words came. Her busy fingers continued to scratch at the tape.

As soon as they exited the room, Jill started grilling the orderly. "How come no one called report?"

"All I know is I was told to bring her. She's been confused. She'll wander off if you don't get her in restraints or have someone sit with her. A neighbor brought her. Found her wandering outside with no coat and only one shoe. Jerry was supposed to call and tell you. The neighbor didn't know of any family."

Then he was gone. Jill put her hands on her hips and glanced up at the clock. It was 2:30. Emergency wasn't supposed to transport any patients between 2:30 and 3:15 to give the second shift time to finish hearing the day shift's report on their patients. She still had an hour's worth of documentation about her patients to write in their charts. She didn't have time for more work.

As she returned reluctantly to the room, she met her bewildered patient standing in the doorway, dress hanging limply from her thin frame. She had succeeded in disconnecting the IV fluids, but the IV catheter was still in her wrist, blood dripping from it freely. Jill was tired, frustrated, and overwhelmed. Her first impulse was to run away from the figure, but instead she gently raised Mrs. Garrison's wrist over her head, grabbed a pair of gloves and walked her back to the bed to begin sorting out the problems that had brought her to the hospital.

The nursing profession is a little like Mrs. Garrison, ailing, uncertain, and a little confused about its future. Though it is understandable why some nurses are turning their backs on the profession and seeking other careers, nursing needs dedicated, flexible, and motivated members now more than ever. It is time for redirection, for nurses to discover that the patient most in need of attention is the profession itself.

THE LEGACY OF FLORENCE NIGHTINGALE

Until now, we have focused on factors outside of nursing and how managed care, hospital executives, regulatory bodies, and even doctors have negatively impacted the nurse's working environment. The nursing shortage has been largely attributed to them, but in this chapter we will study the internal features of nursing that have affected the profession adversely. We will consider how nurses have perpetuated the less desirable traits of the profession and, more important, what they can do to lift the profession to a new level of respect, pride, and honor that will make everyone wish they could experience what it means to be a nurse. For a deeper understanding of the issues facing nursing from within, it is vital to consider how nursing as a profession evolved.

Modern nursing has its roots in the teachings of a dedicated, fierce, and tireless woman named Florence Nightingale, who gained prominence after she was dispatched to the site of the Crimean War in 1854 to care for the wounded British soldiers. What she found in the military hospital was abject filth sprinkled with lice and rats. Her focus and that of the thirty-eight women who accompanied her became cleaning: the floors, the beds, the linens, the kitchen, the water supply system, the men's bodies, and anything that came into contact with them. Mortality rates dropped dramatically. Nursing was born.

Ms. Nightingale was the first to establish nursing as a profession separate from medicine. She saw nursing as a moral imperative, a natural outgrowth of female responsibility, and she devoted her life to the caring of others. She turned down at least two marriage proposals, stating that marriage and the satisfaction she might derive would distract her from her mission. The contribution she made to women of that era cannot be overstated. Women who had no means of independent support and no male to support them were considered a burden on British society, but given an honorable profession, women were effectively emancipated. They could earn an income independently. Though she liberated women on the one hand, she constrained them on the other by insisting that only men should be doctors and that nurses should defer to their authority.

The relative position and delegated gender of nurses and doctors is a concept that grew out of the times in which Ms. Nightingale lived and as such should be left behind by nursing. Fully half of the students entering medical school today are women and are equally good physicians as men. The men who have entered nursing, though far fewer in number, are equally good nurses as the women. And the best patient outcomes occur when both professions work side by side, sharing their knowledge and expertise, rather than one above the other.

Knowledge of disease and medicine has also progressed tremendously since the 1800s, and with it the care that is required. Ms. Nightingale emphasized the patient's physical environment as the focus of nursing tasks. It is known now, however, that while sanitary conditions are necessary to promote health, it is only one small part of a complex process. Creating a genuinely healing environment requires that the nurse understand and appreciate the patient's diagnosis, potential complications, and appropriate treatment interventions along with the social framework within which the patient lives. To accomplish this task requires not only education and training, but that the nurse apply strong critical thinking skills to each unique patient situation.

THE DIMINISHING ROLE OF SELF-SACRIFICE

Ms. Nightingale's tireless devotion to the service of others and her demand that the nurses serving under her exhibit the same quality remains a value of modern nursing, a legacy to which nurses continue to aspire. While the nursing profession thrives in an atmosphere of service and dedication, however, it does not require individual self-sacrifice to be effective. Helping others achieve health is not synonymous with denying one's own health. To be truly effective requires that nurses be attuned to their own needs as well as the needs of the patients they serve. Whether the misappropriation of the concept of self-sacrifice by nursing can be attributed to Ms. Nightingale or whether it developed in the times that followed, it has clearly outlived its social usefulness. Certainly, as employers, hospitals have benefited, yet it may be the nurses themselves who help perpetuate the outdated notion of self-sacrifice, while at the same time resenting it.

As a nursing student, I rotated through a busy children's unit, where it was often a challenge to take meal breaks. Nurses expressed an odd ambivalence about it. It was both a badge of martyrdom and a source of much complaining.

"It's so busy here. We hardly ever get to take a lunch," the nurses would tell us, implying that the same was expected of us.

I noticed one nurse, however, who had an equal assignment to the others and appeared very dedicated, but who consistently took thirty minutes out of her day to put up her feet and eat lunch. When I mentioned it to two other RNs, one nodded and agreed that Carol was very efficient. But the second nurse sniffed and added, "Yes, Carol is very good at taking care of herself." And then they shared knowing looks and nudged each other. The message was clear. A *real* nurse ignored her own body's need for nutrition in favor of tending to patient needs, even if they weren't immediate. And by continually sending that message out to any new nurses that entered their unit, the nurses were able to perpetuate their own myth—that good care required abnegation of self.

But is this the impression that nurses intend to foster? Isn't nursing really about care? In the words of Virginia Henderson, a well-known nursing theorist, the nurse's role is "to assist the individual, sick or well, in the performance of those activities contributing to health or its recovery (or to a peaceful death) that he would perform unaided if he had the necessary strength . . . this aspect of her work, that part of her function, she initiates and controls; of this she is the master."[1] This does not sound like a person who either abnegates self or allows herself to be victimized by others.

NURSE VERSUS NURSE

The passive-aggressive, hypercritical behavior that some nurses exhibit in the workplace has been attributed in literature to a syndrome of the oppressed, of people who are held "in their place" by others. Suzanne Gordon and Bernice Buresh report in their book *From Silence to Voice* that when nurses are asked to describe their work, they frequently are self-disparaging, often crediting someone else's role for a positive patient outcome.[2] Their fear of speaking about their work is partly the result of having their work discounted for years, often by the very group with whom they work most closely, physicians. But part of it also results from the behavior of the nurses around them. If one dares to raise her voice, she is somehow betraying the self-effacing character of the profession[3] and if doctors or outsiders don't chastise her, other nurses will. But while the source can be traced and the reaction is explainable, it serves neither the individual nor the profession. This model of nurse as long-suffering, angry victim has no place in today's workforce. For more than a century nurses have been advocating for their patients. Now they need to begin advocating for themselves and each other.

In the survey I distributed at the Infusion Nurses Society, I asked three questions about nurses themselves. I asked if they felt respected by other nurses, to which 126 of 129 responded a definitive yes or usually. To the second question, whether they felt supported by other nurses, 169 responses were given: 40 said no, 44 said yes, and another

85 said sometimes. Many comments were written in, including "Nurses are their own worst enemies"; "Nurses eat their young"; "We would have a big voice if we realized what we offer as a group"; "Nurses spend too much time back-biting"; and "We need to advocate for ourselves." Nine people wrote that they were "tired of so many negative, complaining nurses," all of which indicates that at least a significant minority of nurses neither view themselves as an empowered group nor trust others in the profession. And their attitude is creating an unpleasant work environment for those around them.

ASSUMING AND SHARING POWER

In many hospitals, staffing levels and forced overtime are issues that need addressing, but hospital CEOs won't be educated to change by nurses who feel powerless to stand up for themselves and instead perpetuate their image as martyr. "As a nurse executive," says Fran Bonardi, RN, MBA, and vice president of nursing at a northeastern hospital, "I am delighted when nurses step forward and make decisions about patient care, their schedules, a policy that needs to be changed, or how to problem solve the fact that two nurses have called in on a given shift on their unit." But she acknowledges that nurses who feel like victims are unlikely to take advantage of opportunities for autonomy. In an October 2001 article in the *Journal of Nursing Administration*, Tim Porter-O'Grady, EdD, RN, says that nurses are still voicing the same complaints they did thirty years ago about "not having a voice, not playing a key role in decision-making."[4] Yet he wonders if all the blame can be placed on the administrators. He says that some of the fault lies with the mindset of nursing. When nurses assume positions of power (as in the case of a nurse-manager role), they use it to make good things happen for the members of their group, but they don't share their power. In other words, the administrator may be willing to shift decision making downward, but if the unit manager is not, the bedside nurse is still without autonomy.

An example might occur during a nurse call to a physician. A novice staff nurse, Bill, notes that his patient appears increasingly lethargic and thinks Dr. Jones should be notified. He returns to the nurses' station to tell the charge nurse. She has known Dr. Jones for many years, has a good working relationship with him, and is often sought by him for information. So instead of having Bill place the call, she gathers from him all the appropriate details of the physical assessment, such as a change in blood pressure or oxygen saturation, and then pages the doctor. When Dr. Jones returns the call, she relays the information, gets an order to increase the IV rate and start the patient on oxygen therapy and then communicates it to Bill. On the face of it, it may seem efficient. After all, Bill can return to the patient while the charge nurse awaits the doctor's call, but she also deprives Bill of a relationship-building opportunity with the physician. If Dr. Jones were speaking with Bill directly, he would have the chance to get to know him and begin to trust not only the charge nurse, but Bill's critical-thinking skills as a nurse. The charge nurse loses an opportunity to mentor Bill in communications and she keeps all the power.

As nurses seek collaborative relationships with physicians, extra attention may need to be focused on the workings of their own teams. Within nursing there exists several levels of preparation: the certified nurse's assistant (CNA), who attends some weeks of training and is tested to earn certification; the licensed practical nurse (LPN), whose training in basic bedside care lasts about one year; the diploma registered nurse (RN), who is trained in a hospital-based program for two to three years; the associate's degree nurse, whose training is in a college setting for two to three years; and the bachelor of science degree nurse (BSN), who attends a college or university for four years. Master of science degree nurses (MSNs) may also work in a clinical setting. An RN is charged with overseeing care, but is frequently supported by LPNs and CNAs. Interestingly, just as the RN complains of not being treated respectfully by physicians and of being shut out of collaboration in care, the LPNs and CNAs and even the lesser-trained RNs sometimes report feeling the same way about their RN leaders. Before convincing doctors of the value of collaborating with them, nurses may have to be attentive to what qualities create collaboration (respectful listening, sharing information, seeking input from all caregivers, empowering others) and demonstrate it within their own work groups.

TEAM SOLUTIONS

In breaking the bonds of the old autocratic ways of practicing nursing and moving into a decentralized model, where the power is shifted to the nurses at the bedside, nurses have to be willing to step into a decision-making role and then also be accountable for the decisions they make. In magnet hospitals, teams of frontline nurses are accountable for practice and work-design issues. They consider the challenges nurses face daily and design better approaches to their daily work.

At the Martha Jefferson Hospital in Virginia, a team of nurses was charged with one of the most challenging aspects of nursing, the practice of floating nurses from their home unit, to which they are usually assigned, to another that is short-staffed. Nurses universally dislike the practice of being pulled from their home units. According to Becky Owen, RN, BSN, "it has been documented that nurses dread floating second only to the death of one's patient while they are in attendance." And indeed, from the reactions of both the nurses who were floated and the units they were floated to, it was obvious that no one liked the arrangement. The team was anxious to find a solution. At the first meeting, they were excited to begin, but ultimately they all arrived at the same sad conclusion: Floating wasn't going away. Though everyone agreed that they disliked it, they had all at one time benefited from having another nurse float to their unit. Since illness and unit vacancies were both unpredictable and outside their control, they agreed that floating would have to be tolerated to ensure that there were enough nurses on all units to meet the goal of exceptional patient care.

The next step was to uncover the qualities that made floating so universally disliked. Their reasons fell into three main categories: service excellence—that either the float nurse or the host unit or both forgot to treat the other with respect and kindness; competence—that the assignment was an inappropriate match of competencies; and workforce issues—that patterns of regular call-ins or perpetual short-staffing appeared or that the floater wasn't privy to all the rules of the host unit.

Once the problems were discovered, the team chose a mission statement, "To improve the process of floating through the establishment and evaluation of an efficient process that defines roles, expectations, and competencies." With assistance from the Human Resources department and research into how other hospitals were handling the issue, they established a policy for their trial period. They determined that the floated nurse should always be given the easiest assignment on the host unit. They designed rules regarding appropriate assignments, such as that nurses inexperienced with cardiac monitors might have to float to the cardiac unit, but they couldn't be assigned to watch monitors. If they were assigned patients that required them, that responsibility had to be coassigned to a host nurse. A buddy system was established so that all floated nurses were assigned a buddy on the host unit to answer their questions and help orient them to the unit. Then they created evaluation forms for both the float staff and the host unit that also served as a reminder about expected behavior. The forms asked for such pertinent data as whether the floater was assigned to a "buddy," whether he was greeted with a smile and thanked at the end of the shift, and whether his assignment was appropriate to his skills. The unit was asked similar questions about the floater. Incentive pay was initiated as compensation for the inconvenience of being floated. Periodically, the evaluations were collected and tabulated. Besides satisfaction, they monitored prevalence by day of the week and unit needing help to determine if there were patterns that needed addressing, such as excessive sick days or lack of staffing. Notably, an improvement in attitude was seen almost instantly.

At their most recent review, the team discovered that 100 percent of the time the float was competency appropriate, the floater's expertise matched the assignment, and 95 percent of the time floaters were assigned a buddy. The result, says Becky Owen, the team's leader, "is that people still aren't happy about having to float, but they are happier floaters." Equally important, the successful working of the float team served as a model for the many teams that followed as the nurses moved toward self-governance.

RESEARCH DEMONSTRATES THE VALUE OF NURSING

Positive portrayals of nurses in the media often touch only on the human interest aspect of their work, the part that is easiest to convey. When it comes to exciting surgical or technical procedures, it is often the physician who stands out as the hero (though the assistance of the nurse is vital). Once the procedure is complete, however, the physician disappears and the patient is left in the capable hands of a nurse. But because a nurse's work is as much about constant observing and assessing as it is about doing, its importance is not always well communicated. It is no wonder that when hospitals were seeking a means of cutting costs, they looked to decreasing their number of nurses. The nonclinical leaders didn't understand the nurses' role and the nurses had no means of quantifying their work in a meaningful way. But nurse researchers are changing that.

Research by advanced-degree nurses is helping the nursing profession establish a new, bolder identity. "Nurse researchers are very interested in trying to document in objective, scientific terms what nurses already know—that nursing care is very important to achieving good patient outcomes," says Linda H. Aiken, PhD, director of the Center for Health Outcomes and Policy Research.[5]

Surveillance and reaction to it are a natural part of a nurse's daily work. Unless there is a problem, it is also a nearly invisible process. The nurse is constantly monitoring and assessing the patient's status for signs of change and either intervenes to prevent a complication or acts quickly as the complication develops to save the patient from a negative consequence, as with Mrs. Garrison, the confused patient. When Nurse Rhodes saw what was happening, she intervened by raising the patient's arm over her head to stop the bleeding while she gathered the necessary supplies to complete the job correctly. That she interceded was so natural to the nurse, she might never have given it another thought. But what if the nurse had not returned immediately to the room? Mrs. Garrison could have gone on losing blood, significantly prolonging and complicating her hospital stay.

In Dr. Aiken's study, as reported in the *American Journal of Nursing*, the researchers were able to quantify nursing surveillance by demonstrating that a lower level of staffing by nurses was correlated to a 7 percent increased risk of death following common surgical procedures.[6] She points out that "the difference in the risk of dying in a hospital in which . . . nurses care for four patients compared to eight patients is near 30 percent." In other words, a nurse's work matters. When a nurse is assigned more (than four) patients and has less time to observe and interact with each, the patient is at a greater risk of dying. Nurses all over the country stood up a little straighter when those study results were announced. She further states that "nurse researchers have placed a high priority on providing very strong evidence of the link between nurse staffing and patient outcomes to give clinical nurses more scientific evidence to argue for improved nurse staffing," signaling that there is more information to come.

Another area to which Dr. Aiken has devoted study is the effect of magnet hospitals on the nurses who work in them and the patients who are admitted. As mentioned in the previous chapter, not only was it demonstrated that magnet hospitals have lower nurse turnover rates, their patients also were shown to have a 4.6 percent lower mortality rate. For the nurses, magnet hospitals are appealing for a number of reasons, including greater autonomy and better collaborative relationships with doctors. Achieving the designation, however, requires both dedication and upfront expense, and some hospitals have resisted. But Dr. Aiken's study gives nurses the evidence they need to prove to hospital CEOs that the hospital ultimately benefits by pursuing magnet status, both financially and in the quality of patient outcomes.

CONTINUING EDUCATION

To assume the autonomous roles and collegial professional relationships that are a hallmark of the magnet program, nurses need a strong commitment to further education. Though for decades it has been diploma and AD nurses who have been the backbone of nursing, in this age of complexity a BSN may become increasingly necessary. At one time, that spelled trouble for AD and diploma nurses. Pursuit of another degree often required that they quit working, an option few adult nurses have, but the climate has changed considerably. Not only are college and universities offering part-time and flexible programs, but technology has brought many other options. Nursing schools offer videoconference classes at remote locations. Others offer low-residency programs where most of the work is done within the nurse's own community with semiannual visits to campus. Still others have once-a-month weekend programs. And online programs are available even for advanced-degree programs. They are no less rigorous than any other program, but online courses are available to students twenty-four hours a day, seven days a week. Nurses can choose to do their class work whenever it fits into their work and home schedule.

Improving one's educational credentials not only helps one gain the respect of others, but helps create more self-confidence and opens up new opportunities. Advanced-degree nurses are in great demand. According to Linda Aiken, "Investigator-initiated nursing research on high-priority research questions central to nursing practice generally requires a doctoral degree at a research-intensive university and, often, postdoctoral research training. Many leading institutions offer full financial support to nurses to pursue doctoral and postdoctoral training. Moreover, the career opportunities in research and faculty positions are immense as the nation is experiencing a severe shortage of nursing faculty." The lack of qualified nursing educators is a major contributor to the nursing shortage. Nursing programs have had to decrease the number of students admitted to their programs because of a lack of qualified professors. Like many nurses, the nursing faculty is aging and a wave of retirements is expected in the next several years. There are fewer graduates from master's and doctoral nursing programs to replace them, and for those who are graduating, higher compensation can be found in clinical positions than in teaching.[7] During the 2000–01 school year nearly six thousand students were turned away from nursing schools because of a shortage of faculty and classroom space. During that same year, 220 schools reported 379 nursing faculty vacancies.[8]

Many employers offer some level of tuition reimbursement to their employees, and as awareness of the shortage heightens, it will likely be offered universally especially for diploma or AD nurses who are willing to get their bachelor's degree. There are even hospitals that agree to forgive the cost of tuition in exchange for a commitment to a certain number of years of future employment. With the advent of the new flexible degree programs and the likelihood of a nurse's employer picking up the cost of the degree, there may be no better time for nurses to return to school for further education.

But continuing education isn't restricted to degree work or a structured classroom. Within the structure of a degree program, it is not possible to keep up with the constant changes in technology and practice. For that, nurses need to regularly attend nursing conferences and meetings and read professional journals. And those things can best be accessed by joining professional organizations. Nursing associations fall into two general categories: specialty nursing groups that focus and disperse information on a specific aspect of nursing practice, and broader general groups that help create the structure within which nursing is practiced. Each is important in its contributions to nursing. The best approach is to maintain membership in both, one group that focuses on the particular specialty area in which a nurse practices and the other a group that considers larger nursing issues.

THE PRESIDENT OF THE ANA SPEAKS OUT

The American Nursing Association is one group that represents the broad scope of nursing. As an organization, it seeks to give nurses a voice in the legislative and regulatory issues that profoundly affect nurses' ability to practice. The ANA lobbied vigorously in support of the Nurse Reinvestment Act, a bill passed by Congress to support nursing education, award scholarships, and forgive tuition for those who earn advanced degrees for teaching, and pledges to continue lobbying for the commitment of the financial support the act will require annually. The ANA journals seek to inform nurses of new and ongoing research, changes in nurse practice, and new legislation that affects all nurses.

As a nurse of eighteen years, I knew little about the American Nursing Association, but in researching the nursing profession for this book, I found myself returning again and again to the ANA Web site, http://nursingworld.org. It is packed with information about nursing, including topics whose importance I had never really understood, such as impending legislation about nursing, recommended criteria for establishing staffing levels, nurse satisfaction surveys, and information about nursing research. Why hadn't I heard more about them? I decided to find out. I called the ANA office, explained my project, and was kindly granted a telephone interview in January 2003 with a very busy woman, Barbara Blakeney, RN, president of ANA. The pride she takes in the profession of nursing, and the passion it incites in her was obvious in the few moments we shared. What follows is a synopsis of our conversation:

Q: *I've been a nurse many years and don't know much about the ANA. Is there a single compelling reason why people should join? How does it benefit nurses in general?*

A: There are many wonderful specialty nurse organizations that help establish the practice of nursing. ANA does the foundational work of the profession; it concentrates on "the work of nursing," not the practice. The ANA pays attention to the infrastructure of nursing; considers impending legislation that may affect us, such as the Nurse Reinvestment Act; monitors the Nurse Practice Acts in each state; and makes sure that the regulatory bodies are properly interpreting quality standards. An organization like the ANA helps create the "house" in which nursing practice happens. We all make a difference as individuals, but joining an association helps us make a difference as part of a larger community. There are lots of ways that nurses take care of people, but who ensures that it can happen? In law, medicine, engineering, there are professional associations that create the infrastructure that makes it possible for their work to occur. Through the American Nurses' Credentialing Center, for instance, we have established the Magnet Recognition program, a structure that hospitals can use to create a better environment for nursing to occur. By joining the ANA, the nurses' dues help us to continue our work on all these fronts.

Q: *Many nurses find it difficult to speak to the media. How did you become so proficient?*

A: Experience. I've made errors, of course, but I've worked with the

ANA on the state level as well as the national level and have served in many different offices and functions. I've had practice and with practice you get better. It's been a wonderful experience. I wouldn't trade it for anything. By working at all levels, I've gained an understanding of the breadth of the profession and worked with many great leaders. I'm thrilled to serve as president.

Q: What about nursing education? What are your recommendations?

A: Never stop learning. Look at the advances, the huge technological explosion in healthcare. You can now swallow a pill that takes pictures and doctors can perform surgery in remote locations via the Internet. We are on the cusp of a scientific revolution. In that environment, nurses can't ever stop learning. We have to look to the future. The educational process will evolve and change as we take dramatic steps forward. The nurses who are practicing now are doing an excellent job, but we will need to continually learn. Things that we accepted as scientific certainties when I started practicing are no longer true.

Q: If you were to advise nurses on just one thing they could do right now to help themselves, what would it be?

A: Be proud to be a nurse!

SPECIALTY NURSES' ORGANIZATIONS

While the associations with broader scope seek to provide the framework for nursing, it is the well-respected specialty nursing associations, such as the Oncology Nurses Society or the Infusion Nurses Society, that develop and advance standards of practice for their specialties. When giving chemotherapy, for instance, it is the Oncology Nurses Society to whom nurses look for the standards by which it is administered. If a nurse has a question about special intravenous lines, she can contact the Infusion Nurses Society for information and standards of practice. Many nursing specialties also offer certifications in their area. The Infusion Nurses Society offers an exam for certification that requires renewal every three years, achievable by either retesting or proof of attendance at approved conferences. Employers frequently offer financial support both for attendance at conferences and for certification. Nurses who work in hospitals that have not historically supported continuing education can request it, correlating it directly to quality of care.

SHARING NURSING KNOWLEDGE

The real value of learning is in sharing knowledge with others. Nurses can share journal articles with other nurses in journal clubs or at staff meetings to enhance the attitude of learning within individual units. New products, new technology, and new methods for giving care are regularly showcased in the nursing journals. There was a time when nurses could graduate from nursing school and expect to practice in the same manner for the rest of their career. Those days are past. Remaining current with the literature and attending educational meetings are an integral part of being a professional and help promote a positive image of nursing to the public. As nurses assume greater pride in their profession, it can't help but have a positive effect on recruitment.

Sharing knowledge with the public gives nurses the opportunity to help the others in their community understand more about vital health issues while also promoting a positive image of nursing. There are so many misconceptions about current health topics. Churches and many civic groups welcome guest speakers whom they feel can offer valuable information to their members. With a little planning and preparation ahead of time, nurses can use their experience to create a presentation related to their specialty. Pediatric nurses, for instance, may want to address common safety hazards for children. Cardiology nurses can talk about the prevention of heart disease and hypertension and give real-life examples of the chronic nature of the disease. Our country is suffering from an epidemic of obesity. Who knows better than nurses about the impact of obesity on health? Nurses can share information on diabetes, chronic lung diseases, and prevention of cancer. Besides taking the opportunity to perhaps discover a previously hidden talent for public speaking, nurses will be presenting the profession in a positive light, as authorities on their topic and as someone others would want to emulate. Schools are great places to share knowledge. Nurses can tell students about what a day in the life of a nurse is really like, the many challenges that are faced and conquered daily.

THE MAGIC STETHOSCOPE *BY R. N. HOPE*

One special group of nurses tapped into their creative writing talent for a unique approach to recruiting and communicating the exciting qualities of a nurse's work to young people. What began as a class exercise in enhancing nurses' writing skills at a George Mason University summer course turned into a book, *The Magic Stethoscope.*[9] Published under the collective pen name of R. N. Hope in November 2002, the book tells of two siblings, aged ten and seven, who find a magic stethoscope in their parents' attic and are whisked off to experience firsthand what it is like to be a nurse. The characters don't think they have any interest in such a career, but both are surprised to learn how much nurses do.

Jeanne Sorrell, PhD, who is the associate dean for academic programs and research at George Mason University's College of Nursing and Health Science, taught the writing class and helped shape the book into a cohesive form by adding a first and last chapter, but the other stories belong to the nurses in the class.

Each chapter of the book shows a different aspect of nursing, based on the real-life experiences of the authors. Because they all came from different backgrounds, the class contributors give a true flavor of the rich variety of jobs that can be found in nursing. They also didn't spare the truth. The first adventure is shocking a man's heart back into regular rhythm in an emergency room. Another involves a kidney transplant with a sister donating her kidney to her ailing twin. A baby is delivered in the back of a taxi and a young victim of trauma is transported from a helicopter bay to emergency care. The intention of the writers was to give middle school–aged children a new vision of the importance of a nurse's work and perhaps inspire some of them to become nurses in the future. Fittingly, proceeds from the sales of the book go into a scholarship fund for nursing at George Mason University.

Dr. Sorrell says that since the *Washington Post* ran Leef Smith's feature on the book in January 2003, it has generated a lot of interest. She has received many inquiries about purchase. Though the book is currently available only through the GMU nursing college, Dr. Sorrell says that distribution will be broadening to Internet sales and is likely to enter a second printing. Arrangements are also being made translate the book into Spanish. Further information including how *The Magic Stethoscope* can be ordered is found on page 221, in appendix F

PORTRAYING A POSITIVE IMAGE

When I was a novice nurse in the mid-1980s, there was a short-lived nursing shortage. Hospitals in the area banded together to promote nursing, visiting high schools and middle schools and giving a press conference for the local media. I was asked by the hospital to speak. I was uncertain about the words that would come out of my mouth until I approached the microphone. So many images came to my mind. I had been working only a couple of years and was still a little uncertain of my skills. Though I usually left work exhausted and lunch was hit-or-miss at best, it was still the best job I had ever had. For all the hardships, I realized that what was most true about being a nurse for me was that every day I left the hospital knowing that I had helped someone, that a patient was a step closer to restored health because of some action I had taken. Most days I couldn't believe that I was so lucky to have found such a perfect profession! If the opportunity of speaking were to arise again, knowing what I do now, I would be more conscious of how I represented the profession, of emphasizing the skill and training that was required for me to help the patients toward wellness, but at the time, my work was a simple, unconscious expression of joy, something that few professions can inspire as profoundly as nursing.

The experience of nursing is rich with stories. Yet nurses as a group are often reluctant to share their stories, especially stories that might feature themselves in some heroic role. In *From Silence to Voice: What Nurses Know and Must Communicate to the Public*, Bernice Buresh and Suzanne Gordon make a good case for nurses being the best providers of information about nursing to the public. They discuss in detail how cultural and historical influences, many of which were gender related, created a professional group so reluctant to talk about themselves and the value of their work. It is a step-by-step guide that helps nurses develop a strong voice for themselves, their patients, and the profession. The authors point out the many self-effacing and self-defeating actions that nurses unwittingly perform each day, from self-introductions that don't include their title and last name to hiding behind the term "we" when speaking of any accomplishment, from denigrating themselves when someone says "thank you" to attributing the credit for a positive patient outcome to someone else. Numerous examples and case studies contribute to a fascinating read that will leave nurses feeling cheered and proud of the work they do. But its first important lesson is in simply formulating and practicing the stories.

At the hospital where I work, we were meeting to create a new mission and vision statement to guide nursing as we prepared for the transition to shared governance. Using *From Silence to Voice* as a stepping stone, nurses were assigned to bring to the meeting a story about someone in nursing who had inspired them. Many of the nurses participated. Telling someone else's story wasn't so hard. After talking about the premise of the book and reading aloud some of the stories it recounted, group members were asked to tell a story of nursing with themselves as the heroes. This proved a much harder assignment. When we came back together, there was initially only silence. Very slowly the stories began to come out, as did the tears, because nurse stories are often touching, capturing people at their most honest and vulnerable moments.

Brenda Welch, RN, BA, CHPN (certified hospice and palliative care nurse), told of her background as a city girl who decided to move to the country to be a hospice nurse. Her first patient was a farmer. Though he knew he was dying, he kept on living, kept on being a farmer until it was his time. She told of making her visits to him and though the time had been prearranged, rather than being at the house he would be out in the field on his tractor. He needed oxygen, so he rigged up a place behind his tractor seat to carry it and wore a mask to keep down the dust. Brenda learned to meet him where he was, to take her stethoscope and blood pressure monitor and walk out into the field. She would ask him to shut off the motor just long enough for her to listen to his heartbeat and then she would ride with him and let him tell her of any difficulties he was having. When he died, it was in his own bed, surrounded by family who sat together sharing stories of his life. It was her care and her willingness to allow him to continue to be himself that helped his death retain the flavor of his life.

Everyone in the room smiled to hear the farmer's story. It's important that nurses let their voices be heard, to share with friends, with the public, or with some potential recruit what it means to be a nurse. Nurses have the power to do more than any other group to ensure that there are enough nurses to meet the needs of American healthcare simply by sharing the truth of the nursing experience.

CREATING A BRIGHTER FUTURE

To ensure a bright future for nursing, the profession itself must continue to assume a strong leadership role. Nurse researchers are helping by providing proof of nursing's vital role in patient care. Nursing associations are empowering their members to seek improved working conditions and better nursing practice models as well as to lead the march toward legislating safe nurse-to-patient ratios. Within their institutions, resourceful nurses are finding their voices and assuming confident, collegial roles as contributing members of interdisciplinary care teams. But there are other, more prickly issues that need to be tackled. Educational requirements for the RN degree may need to become uniform. To earn desired professional respect and to learn the skills needed in the increasingly complex world of healthcare, consideration may have to be given to making the bachelor's degree mandatory for future entry-level nurses. The aim of advanced degree programs may also require a new vision. Rather than earning a nurse a role distanced from the patient, further education could reward the nurse with the opportunity to mentor less-experienced nurses by working alongside them at the bedside. For nowhere in nursing can great leadership earn more intrinsic rewards than in providing direct care to the patient.

NOTES

1. Bernice Buresh and Suzanne Gordon, *From Silence to Voice: What Nurses Know and Must Communicate to the Public* (Ottawa, Ont.: Canadian Nurses Association, 2000), p. 36.

2. Ibid., pp. 31–45.

3. Ibid.

4. Tim Porter-O'Grady, "Is Shared Governance Still Relevant?" *JONA* 31, no. 10 (2001): 468–73.

5. E-mail communication with author, January 27, 2003.

6. Sean P. Clarke and Linda H. Aiken, "Failure to Rescue," *American Journal of Nursing* 103, no.1 (January 2003): 46.

7. "Nursing Faculty Shortage Fact Sheet," American Association of Colleges of Nursing [online] www.aacn.nche.edu/Media/Backgrounders/faculty-shortage.htm [March 28, 2003].

8. Larry Cooper, "The Nursing Shortage: From Bad to Worse," *Hematology Oncology* 1, no. 9 (October 2002): 19.

9. Leef Smith, "An Urgent Message in Nurses' Tale," *Washington Post*, Virginia Extra, January 23, 2003, p. 1.

CHAPTER NINE
Accountability for Health
IT'S NOT JUST FOR
HEALTHCARE PROVIDERS

Hospitals, administrators, doctors, and the nursing profession itself have contributed to the current nursing shortage, but what about the public? As vital as nurses are to patients, are the demands of the public impacting the profession's ability to meet their needs?

Due in large part to the aging baby boomers, the need for nurses is projected to be 26 percent higher in 2010 than it was in 2000. That is the equivalent of nearly half a million nurses. Certainly from the perspective of those involved in healthcare, conditions for nurses are improving as awareness increases and legislators and industry come to the aid of the profession. But even with every hospital becoming a magnet hospital, every workplace becoming a center for collaborative and autonomous partnerships, and every nurse lavishly appreciated every day, would it really be possible to add enough nurses to accommodate the impending need?

During the 1990s, as the cost of healthcare threatened to outstrip the economy's ability to accommodate it, managed care surged to the forefront. It did what its name implies. It sought to "manage" the amount of healthcare used by establishing rules and shifting the providers toward more economical drugs, diagnostic testing, and treatments when the outcome was likely to be the same as when more expensive procedures were used. By 2001 managed care was relaxing its grip on the healthcare economy in the face of the threat of legal and financial consequences for its restrictions. At the same time, the cost of medical care in the United States went up 8.7 percent, the largest rise in more than a decade.[1] The total spending on healthcare represented 14.1 percent of the gross domestic product, the highest percentage in American history.[2] The price tag was not just the result of a rising cost of services, as it sometimes was in the past, but to an increase in the quantity consumed. Spending averaged $5,035 per person.[3]

Some of 2001's increased spending can be explained by the needs of the aging population and the increased costs hospitals have experienced related to wage hikes resulting from worker shortages. But how much of the added cost is due to the lack of responsibility Americans feel toward their own health? Information abounds about the risks of smoking. A warning has been printed on the side of every package of cigarettes for decades, yet millions of Americans continue to smoke. The dangers of eating foods high in saturated fats and the value of eating at least five servings per day of fruits and vegetables is another commonly known fact, yet obesity is quickly becoming the predominant preventable health issue in the country. And both smoking and obesity lead to innumerable health complications that require intervention from nurses.

JENNY'S STORY

Jenny Green* is visiting her doctor for a checkup. He notes that her weight is up by twenty pounds since the previous year's checkup, that her blood pressure is elevated, her cholesterol is up, and her blood sugar seems high. He tells her she is too young for these problems and needs to lose weight. He gives her a prescription for blood pressure medication and signs a lab slip so that she can go to the hospital for further testing for diabetes. Jenny leaves the office. She is in a hurry. She missed her lunch to go for her doctor's appointment, it is nearly time to pick up her youngest from day care, and she is feeling starved. She

---

*Jenny Green is fictional, though the challenges she faces are real.

drives to a fast-food chain, orders from the window, and accepts the suggestion to upgrade the size of her meal. She doesn't bother with a diet drink; she needs the sugar high to get her through the rest of the day. Besides, she can worry about her weight later.

Considering all the factors pressuring Jenny, her choice is understandable. Her doctor told her the one bit of news she least wanted to hear, she had to sacrifice her lunch hour to see him, and then had to wait so long that she couldn't even return to the office. Instead it was time to start her round of afternoon responsibilities: picking up kids, supervising homework, and planning a meal. Then, of course, there was the young man in the drive-thru window who offered for pennies more to double the size of her serving of french fries. Events were conspiring to lead Jenny astray. But understanding why it happened doesn't change the facts. If Jenny doesn't change her habits, she will be greatly increasing her risk of premature death or of contracting a chronic disease that will drain her family's resources. And it won't be the doctor, the fast food server, or her office that will pay the price. It will be Jenny and her family.

Try This Quiz with Jenny (answers appear on page 162):

1. What percentage of Americans are overweight or obese?

    a. 40%
    b. 35%
    c. 50%
    d. 65%

2. What risk could Jenny face if she allows her blood pressure to stay elevated?

    a. stroke
    b. congestive heart failure
    c. both of the above

3. What condition could potentially bankrupt healthcare?
   a. cancer
   b. heart disease
   c. obesity
   d. high blood pressure

4. What percentage of the total healthcare bill in 2001 was spent on chronic diseases whose prevalence could be decreased with preventive action?
   a. 90%
   b. 20%
   c. 75%
   d. 30%

5. What was the total American healthcare bill for 2001?
   a. $125 billion
   b. $30 billion
   c. $60 billion
   d. $1.4 trillion

6. Each year smoking kills more people than:
   a. AIDS
   b. alcohol and drug abuse
   c. car crashes
   d. murders and suicide
   e. all of the above combined

7. If Jenny had a sudden desire to "run off" her double cheeseburger meal, she would need to:
   a. vacuum for an hour
   b. walk briskly on her treadmill for 30 minutes
   c. take a 10-minute stroll around the block
   d. run two-and-a-half hours at a 10-minute-mile pace

The Surprising Answers

Jenny is not alone. Apparently, all over America a variation of the above scene is replayed millions of times a day. In response to the release of the latest statistics about soaring healthcare costs in America, Tommy G. Thompson, the secretary of the Department of Health and Human Services, said that he was determined to "persuade Americans to change their lifestyles."[4] This came in response to the announcement just days before that healthcare spending in America had risen 8.7 percent to $1.4 trillion dollars annually.[5] According to Thompson, 75 percent was spent on the treatment of chronic diseases, many of which can be prevented through healthier lifestyle choices.

In a related story that appeared on CBS News on December 31, 2002, the Centers for Disease Control and Prevention reported that obesity rates had increased from 19.8 percent in 2000 to 20.9 percent in 2001. At the same time the rate of Type II diabetes increased from 7.3 percent to 7.9 percent of the population. There is a strong correlation between obesity and type II diabetes. In April 2003 the American Cancer Society reported that there is also a close relationship between obesity and cancer, following a study that evaluated more than nine hundred thousand people. It concluded that excess body weight was related to 14 percent of cancer deaths in men and 20 percent in women.[6] Obesity is also associated with heart disease, high blood pressure, osteoarthritis, sleep apnea, asthma, gall bladder disease, and depression.[7]

More than 65 percent of Americans are either overweight or obese. Obesity is defined as being roughly thirty pounds or more over one's healthy weight, and overweight is about ten to thirty pounds above a healthy weight.

THE BODY MASS INDEX AS INDICATOR OF OBESITY

The most accurate test of obesity as predictor of health risk is the Body Mass index (BMI). A BMI between 25 and 29.9 is considered overweight. It implies an increased level of health risk, but a BMI over 30 is considered obese and the health risk is much greater. The real formula is based on metric measurements, but the American Obesity Association offers a modification to the formula so that it can be used without converting to metrics. It is necessary to have an accurate height and weight:

$$\text{weight} \div \text{height}^2 \times 704.5 = \text{BMI}$$

Since Tommy Thompson publicly declared his weight, we can use him as an example. He didn't announce his height, so a height of six feet will be assigned to him. Six feet equals seventy-two inches. Squaring (multiplying it by itself) his height would equal 5184. His weight before losing was 215. Divide that by 5184 (his height squared) and then multiply by 704.5.

Tommy Thompson's BMI, prior to weight loss, was 29.2, on the upper edge of the overweight category, nearing obesity. He reported in January of 2003 that he had already lost eighteen pounds (giving him a BMI of 26.7) and that his goal weight was 185. At 185, he will be at a healthy BMI of 25!

The American Obesity Association warns that the formula may be misleading for very muscular people or pregnant women. To have your BMI calculated for you, visit the association's Web site at www.obesity.org.

THE MONETARY COSTS OF OBESITY

Obesity—a largely preventable condition—cost the United States about $123 billion in 2001, according to Anne Wolf of the University of Virginia, as reported in *USA Today*.[8] That figure includes the direct and indirect costs for diseases related to obesity and loss of worker productivity. Obesity's direct costs, according to Wolf, are 30 percent higher than those for coronary heart disease.[9] In the same story, another researcher was quoted as saying that at the current rate, nearly everyone would be overweight by the year 2030. Worse, treatment of the resultant diseases, particularly diabetes, could bankrupt the healthcare system.[10]

Nursing is directly impacted by an increasingly obese population in two ways. Overweight and obese people are more likely than normal-weight individuals to need medical and nursing care, and nurses caring for larger patients are at an increased risk of injury from lifting. Though assistive lifting devices help, they are not always available when unexpectedly needed, such as when a hospitalized patient suddenly feels faint, perhaps having walked to the bathroom and finding herself too weak to get back to bed. In a survey of nurses regarding their safety concerns in the workplace, 60 percent indicated that their greatest fear was a disabling back injury.[11] Since the age of the average nurse is the mid-forties, such injuries become especially problematic.

Curiously, if most Americans were asked, they could recite the causes of obesity, much like Jenny Green, even as they sit next to the drive-thru window. Healthy eating and exercise as a means of controlling weight are words that almost anyone could recite if prompted. The problem lies not only in the gap between knowing and acting, but also in the ways our lives have been altered by technology.

THE PRICE OF PROGRESS

One hundred years ago, when the life expectancy was closer to fifty, Americans labored to make a living and to raise food. Transportation was a pair of shoes. To attend church, school, or work, people often walked or went by horse and carriage. But even a carriage ride was no simple process, requiring that the horse be bridled and hitched to the wagon, and on return be groomed and fed. In between, the stalls had to be cleaned and hay grown for feed. A ride required work! But as personal cars and public transportation became common, people no longer had to expend effort and calories for transportation. Indoor plumbing meant no longer carrying water to the house, and gas and electric stoves preempted the need to cut and chop wood. Jobs changed as well. Jobs featuring manual labor decreased in number, replaced by service or desk work. Still, Americans enjoyed outdoor recreation, in hiking, biking, camping, and playing ball. Then came the television, which slowly ate into outdoor time, followed by remote controls, computers, and video games. Soon the only energy that needed to be expended was walking from the house to the car and from the car to the office or school.

Americans stopped moving, but they didn't stop eating. In fact, they ate just as much, but the nature of the food changed. At the turn of the century, overeating meant eating too many potatoes. Sugar was not a normal part of the diet (about five pounds per year per person). Americans now consume about 170 pounds of sugar annually and drink more soda than water, on average one and a half cans—roughly two hundred and thirty calories—per day.[12] And they eat far too few vegetables. One problem with the consumption of easy-to-fix prepackaged foods is that they often are lacking in fiber, and fiber is what makes a person feel full. An associated problem is what dieticians refer to as "portion distortion." A healthy-sized portion looks too small, in part because large quantities of processed foods can be consumed without a feeling of fullness and in part because the large portion is something that is perpetuated in the media and advertising. Slender people are shown consuming sodas, chocolate, and fried fatty foods. The implication is that the observer also can eat those types of foods in that amount without suffering the consequences. Clearly, however, Americans are suffering the consequences.

THE REAL COST OF FAST FOOD ISN'T JUST THE PRICE

As an example, an average fast food meal can be examined. After consuming a double cheeseburger, large fries, and twenty-four-ounce soda, Jenny feels satisfied. She probably had breakfast, and a few hours after eating the cheeseburger she might sit down to dinner. But the calories in the meal described are the equivalent of what most women need for an entire day, around fifteen hundred calories, and offer little useful nutrition.

A translation of activity into calories can help illustrate the level of distortion that exists concerning the food/fuel relationship. To work off the calories of one small cookie, ten minutes of brisk walking is required, but if the cookie is exchanged for the large gourmet-size cookie more commonly sold individually, that walk continues for another thirty to thirty-five minutes. A jelly donut requires at least an hour. And that fast food meal? The equivalent of fifteen miles; Jenny would need to either run for two and a half hours at a ten-minute-mile pace or spend several hours walking to expend the calories from her lunch. Not many Americans are participating in such an exercise program. In fact, less than a third of adults exercise thirty to forty-five minutes a day, the amount required to maintain good health, and 40 percent do not participate in any formal exercise at all.

OBESITY AND DIABETES

Diabetes is one of the most significant long-term results of obesity. It is a condition in which the body doesn't produce enough of the hormone insulin. Insulin helps glucose (sugar) move into the body's cells, where it is needed for fuel. If there isn't enough insulin or if it is ineffective, the level of glucose in the circulating blood stays high. The cells are then starved for fuel and the blood sugar levels can begin to damage nerves and blood vessels, which leads to heart disease. It is the small vessels that are particularly vulnerable, however, producing such complications as blindness, kidney failure, and diminishing feeling in the legs and feet. Amputation of toes, feet, or legs result from the decreasing circulation and nerve injury in the lower extremities. Avoiding refined sugars becomes especially important to diabetics to help control blood sugar levels. After eating, the body begins to convert the food into glucose for fuel. Foods such as vegetables contain healthy fiber, which slows the conversion and allows the glucose to be gradually added to the circulating blood. Starchy foods that have higher concentrations of sugar are converted a little faster, but refined sugar hits the blood stream all at once, causing an immediate spike that is difficult to control.

Type I diabetes (not known to be preventable) most often appears in childhood or adolescence because the body can't produce enough insulin. In Type II diabetes, however, the body makes insulin, but doesn't use it effectively. It has historically been a disease that is diagnosed after age forty, when the most extra body weight tends to accumulate, but due to increasing rates of childhood obesity and lack of exercise, Type II diabetes is appearing even in children.[13] (Since 43 percent of adolescents watch more than two hours of television each day, there is little time left for movement.)[14]

Obesity and Mobility

Another affliction associated with obesity is osteoarthritis. During mobility, it is the joints that allow for flexion (bending) and the long muscles of the legs that do much of the work. If leg muscles are allowed to weaken due to lack of use, the joints have to take on more of the work with less support from the surrounding muscles. Add extra weight and the strain on the joints becomes even greater. The cartilage in the joints becomes worn and little cushion remains between the bones. The result is pain and inflammation. Even modest weight loss can help relieve the symptoms and delay progression of the disease.

As a new nurse, I cared for an older woman who was in the hospital for hip replacement surgery. She had a difficult postoperative period and because she was quite obese, there wasn't always enough manpower to assist her. One morning, as she was laboring to take a step with her walker, I asked when she would be returning for the second surgery. She said not until her first replacement was pain free and wondered aloud if that would ever happen. I asked gently if her physician had ever suggested that weight loss might take some of the pressure off her joints and reduce her pain. She looked very surprised that I should ask. I didn't see her again until six months later when she returned to have the other hip replaced. She recuperated from the second procedure much more quickly than the first. She had lost thirty pounds due to a gastrointestinal complication, and although she was still categorized as obese her weight loss had made a remarkable difference in the speed of her recovery. She was so inspired by her success that she began an intentional diet and lost an additional fifty pounds. When I last saw her she reported feeling twenty years younger.

Obesity and High Blood Pressure

High blood pressure, a silent threat, has a very high correlation with extra body weight. More than 75 percent of hypertension cases can be directly attributed to obesity.[15] Combined with age, it is the strongest indicator of the condition. Unfortunately, since high blood pressure is largely without symptoms until it is too late, it can be ignored without regular checkups. Left untreated, it can progress to stroke or congestive heart failure. Heart disease, which can lead to heart attack, sudden cardiac arrest, chest pain, and abnormal heart rhythm, is also more common in persons who are overweight or obese.

Extra weight stored as fat overburdens many of the body's systems and interferes with proper functioning. The American Obesity Association listed six pages of medical conditions either caused by or closely associated with obesity. In addition to those mentioned, obesity can contribute to gout, difficulty healing, heat intolerance, breathlessness, and body pain.

JENNY'S CHOICE

Jenny Green has choices. She is suffering high blood pressure and appears to be a borderline diabetic, but if she decides to alter her habits even slightly, she can improve her health. If not, her outlook is less favorable.

Jenny decides to do nothing. She fills her prescription for blood pressure medication and takes it when she remembers. She doesn't like the side effects, though, the tiredness and the diminished libido. Her doctor also prescribes medication to control her blood sugar levels.

By the time she is forty years old, Jenny is in the hospital with dizziness and hypertension. Her blood sugar is out of control. She is five-foot-five and 270 pounds. Her doctor thinks it is time for her to begin giving herself shots of insulin, since the pills are no longer effective. Her nurse spends time with her teaching her about the diabetes and how her obesity, diabetes, and hypertension put her at a very high risk of stroke. During her stay, Jenny gets up to the bathroom and has a syncopal (fainting) episode. Her nurse is with her and tries to catch her to prevent her from hitting the floor. Jenny is fine, but the nurse misses three weeks of work from a resulting back injury.

Before she is fifty, Jenny is hospitalized three more times—twice related to her diabetes and once from a wrenched disc she suffers while vacuuming. Each incident requires extensive nursing care. At fifty-two,

Jenny has a stroke. She is rushed by ambulance to the hospital. Her heart stops beating on the way and CPR is begun. She remains on life support in the intensive care unit for two days while the family agonizes over what they should do. Finally, her distraught husband agrees that she would not want to continue in a vegetative state and allows the nurses to remove her from the ventilator. Jenny dies three months before her younger daughter's wedding.

THE COST OF SMOKING

Smoking is another lifestyle choice that can cause preventable conditions that significantly impact health and well-being. Smoking-related diseases kill more than four hundred thousand Americans each year, more than AIDS, alcohol, drug abuse, car accidents, murders, and suicides combined.[16] The direct medical costs amount to more than $50 billion a year in the United States. Until obesity surged to the forefront, smoking was associated with the highest preventable costs in healthcare.

In conjunction with obesity, smoking is especially potent. Each condition contributes to heart disease, elevated blood pressure, elevated blood sugar, and damaged nerves and kidneys. Together they pack an extra punch.

To most smokers, none of the above is news. Since the 1960s a label has been added to each pack of cigarettes warning of its potential for harm. Yet it is difficult to give up. Nicotine, the drug found in tobacco, is highly addictive. For those who smoke regularly, stopping can bring on physical withdrawal symptoms such as headaches, irritability, sweating, constipation, or diarrhea. It is often worse on the second day after quitting and takes time to disappear entirely. Even harder for some people are the psychological aspects of smoking. Much like overeaters do with eating, smokers attach many positive associations to the act of smoking. For many, it is the first thing to do upon awakening or the last thing to do before going to sleep, and it provides a means of relaxation and comfort at any point in the day.

But death by cigarettes is often a slow suffocation. With emphysema in its end stages, for example, any movement, even as simple as brushing teeth or walking to the bathroom, results in breathlessness, a struggle for oxygen. A lung cancer patient I once took care of summed it up best. It was in the late 1980s, when patients and visitors to hospitals could still smoke. I was treating a man in his late fifties with chemotherapy for his lung cancer. It was his third cycle of drugs and his veins had gotten scarce. I was having a difficult time finding one that would accept an intravenous catheter needle and the man had developed a phobia of sharp things. On my third attempt, while he cringed and gritted his teeth, I finally was able to start the IV. I reviewed the side effects of the drugs with him and pretreated for nausea. His nephew sat in the corner of the room, chain-smoking. They made small talk while I continued to administer the drugs. Finally unable to contain myself, I asked the younger man if his uncle's fate had made him consider quitting. "Nah," he said. "We all have to go somehow." Just about then, his uncle's IV began to infiltrate into the surrounding tissues. I had to pull the needle and begin a new search for a willing vein. As the needle was unsheathed, revealing the sharp tip, the older man grimaced and pulled back involuntarily. He closed his eyes and leaned back on the pillow, holding himself rigid. "We may all have to go, son, but I bet there's easier ways."

UNCOVERING THE CAUSE

No dollar figure can adequately measure the personal tragedy suffered by Jenny and her family or by the man with lung cancer. Lifestyle-related chronic disease creates a significant emotional impact on personal lives. It also creates a drain on public healthcare resources, including nurses. That raises an important question: Why haven't lifestyle habits changed? For instance, 61 percent of Type II diabetes, which can lead to loss of limbs and eyesight, is directly linked to obesity.[17] Healthier diets and increased exercise could greatly reduce the number of cases diagnosed, yet Americans grow more obese with each passing year.

Is it possible that the public doesn't believe that there is a relationship between lifestyle and health, or is it simply that they have the unrealistic expectation that modern healthcare can undo whatever harm they inflict? It is easy to understand how either misconception could exist. The public is bombarded daily with advertisements for hospitals that claim the ability to save people from heart disease or cancer. Nightly television magazines masquerading as news programs often showcase medical advances as miraculous. People within the medical field itself perpetuate the myth by not always sharing the whole truth about research results, new medications and treatments, or even a patient's prognosis. Then there are the advertisements, television shows, and movies that show slender, healthy people gulping fatty, fried foods, drinking sugar-laden sodas and alcohol, and smoking cigarettes as if their habits are without consequence. No wonder expectations are inflated out of proportion.

Along with misplaced expectations, however, there is another culprit in lifestyle-related illnesses: the refusal to acknowledge personal responsibility for our actions. Just as juvenile violence is blamed on gun makers, video games, movies, and music rather than the poor choices of the young individual, overeating is blamed on the fast-food industry and smoking on the tobacco industry rather than the person who chooses to overeat or light a cigarette. But to make changes, the power and the responsibility has to be returned to the individual. The addiction doesn't simply disappear. The person struggling with it has to make a decision to take an action to get help in fighting it.

Regardless of why the warnings about the association between lifestyle and health are ignored, there is no denying that habits such as smoking and overeating increase the quantity of healthcare needed. As there is already a shortage of nurses to give that care, it becomes especially important that American lifestyles are modified to avoid preventable health conditions. The aging population will challenge healthcare in the future, but if lifestyle-related diseases of the proportions currently projected flood the healthcare system at the same time, the result may be that no one receives the quality care they deserve, because there won't be enough nurses to fill the need.

Another area in which the public's active role can help nursing is in the creation of advance directives. There are times when doctors and nurses are forced to administer aggressive treatment even in the face of almost certain death because the patient has not indicated beforehand under what conditions he would prefer to be administered comfort measures rather than active treatment. In the following chapter, the patient's right to choose and the laws that protect that right will be discussed.

NOTES

1. Robert Pear, "Spending on Health Care Increased Sharply in 2001," *New York Times* [online], www.nytimes.com/2003/01/08/health/08HEAL. html [January 8, 2003].

2. Ibid.

3. Katharine Levit et al., "Trends in U.S. Health Care Spending, 2001," *Health Affairs* 22, no. 1 (January/February 2003): 154.

4. Robert Pear, "Emphasize Disease Prevention, Health Secretary Tells Insurer," *New York Times* [online]. www.nytimes.com/2003/01/22/politics/ 22HEAL.html [January 21, 2003].

5. Pear, "Spending on Health Care Increased Sharply in 2001."

6. Associated Press, "Study Hailed as Convincing in Tying Fat to Cancers," *New York Times* [online], www.nytimes.com/2003/04/24/health [April 24, 2003].

7. "The Surgeon General's Call to Action to Prevent and Decrease Overweight and Obesity," Virtual Office of the Surgeon General [online], www.surgeongeneral.gov/topics/obesity/ calltoaction/fact_consequences.htm [January 2003].

8. Nanci Hellmich and Anita Mannng, "Scales Tiping toward Diabetes: Twin Scourge of Weight and Disease Could 'Break the Bank' of Healthcare," *USA Today*, October 24, 2003. This article is no longer archived at the *USA Today site*, but it is available at www.defeatdiabetes.org/Articles/obesity3021024.htm.

9. Ibid.

10. Ibid.

11. "Health & Safety Survey," Nursing World [online], http://nursing-world.org/surveys/hssurvey/pdf [September 2001].

12. "Eating Low-Fat and Still Gaining—How?" Oregon Health Sciences University [online], www.ohsu.edu/som-lipid/vol133/sugar.htm [November 3, 1998].

13. "Your Weight and Diabetes," North American Association for the Study of Obesity [online], www.naaso.org/information/diabetes_obesity.asp [January 2003].

14. "The Surgeon General's Call to Action," Virtual Office of the Surgeon General.

15. "Health Effects of Obesity," American Obesity Association [online], www.obesity.org/subs/fastfacts/Health_Effects.shtml [February 2003].

16. "Smoking Statistics," *Advance for Nurses* 4, no. 16 (August 5, 2002): 46.

17. Hellmich and Manning, "Scales Tipping toward Diabetes."

Answers to the quiz on pp. 149–50.

1. d, 2. c, 3. c. 4. c, 5. d, 6. e, and 7. d.

CHAPTER TEN
Advance Directives
COMMUNICATING YOUR WISHES

As discussed in earlier chapters, medical advances have turned many once-fatal conditions into merely chronic ones, increasing the need for nursing care. At the same time, the definitions of life and death have grayed, creating difficult ethical dilemmas for nurses, especially in critical-care areas. At what point does help become harm? Some might contend that life after resuscitation has meaning only if the person is restored to his condition prior to needing medical intervention. In other words, if the person has both physical and cognitive functions intact. Someone else may define life much more broadly consider meaningful life to exist as long as by any mechanism oxygen can be circulated through the body, even if only by machine. Death was once as simple as one's breath ceasing and the heart no longer beating, but in recent decades, with the advent of resuscitation, some small prospect exists for a second chance, giving family, significant others, and the healthcare team the terrible burden of making a choice.

Mike Berry* is from healthy stock, a physical kind of man who loves the outdoors. At sixty-nine, he still kayaks, hikes, and bikes in the summer. During the long winter months, he traipses through the woods on

---

*Mike Berry and the other characters in this chapter are fictitious, though the challenges they face are real.

snowshoes when conditions are right, but otherwise he putters around the house, repairing leaking faucets and squeaky floorboards and waiting for the days to grow longer. His wife is content to stay home and read, but she always knows when the sap is rising. By the end of February, Mike is prowling the house like a caged animal, waiting for the ice to leave the waterways. On an afternoon in mid-March when the temperature is nearing fifty degrees, he takes a drive, wandering the back roads and winding up at the old bridge that crosses Putnam Creek. The water has quickened since his last visit and the ice floes are piling up in the sycamore grove on the other side of the creek. He can feel the rush in his veins, sensing that spring is near, that soon he'll be back in the water, negotiating the rapids on the south side of the bridge. He cranes his neck to see over the side of the railing, and then he notes movement from his left side, a young boy on a bike. Startled, he slams on his brakes, catches some ice under his wheel, and starts to spin. Minutes after the boy calls 911, Mike is pulled from the icy waters. Two rescue workers try to revive him as he is rushed to the hospital. When his wife arrives, she finds her husband with a tube down his throat and a ventilator breathing for him. A monitor screen shows the blips of his heartbeat. The doctor tells her that he may never awaken, that the machine is breathing for him, and that if they take him off he will be unable to continue on his own. What does she want the medical team to do?

Hilda Sanford enters the hospital for her hip replacement surgery. She is cheerful going in, not looking forward to the surgery but anxious to be back on her feet as she awaits the birth of her first grandchild. She is approaching fifty, young for joint replacement, but it will repair a congenital anomaly that has plagued her for years. A plump little woman with soft pink cheeks and eyes creased with a thousand smiles, she is relieved when the surgery is over. The hip is painful, but she is anxious to begin rehabilitation. Her goal is to be free of any assistive devices before her grandbaby arrives. She can't wait to see him. On her third postoperative day, the evening nurse walks in to say good night and discovers her skin is cool to the touch. She is not breathing. The nurse calls a code. When her husband rushes back to the hospital thirty minutes later, they are still working on her.

What would Mike Berry want his wife to do? And what about Hilda Sanford and her husband? Guesses can be made, but without a living will or an advance directive to guide families and the healthcare team toward the next step, the decision can be very difficult.

Thirty years ago, it would have been simpler. Both patients would have died. Now the boundaries are not so simple. People in hospitals no longer die, they "code." When a patient is found lifeless, a code is called and an emergency team comes rushing. The team may pump the patient full of drugs to stimulate the heart and apply paddles to the chest, sending volts of electricity through the body. They may intubate the patient, placing a tube down his throat, and place him on a venti-lator that will breathe for him. Sometimes these steps are taken because there is a genuine hope of recuperation and other times it is a rote motion to preempt the possibility of a lawsuit.

For nurses, who are the usual initiators, running a code can be emo-tionally devastating not simply because of the life that may be lost, but because the purpose for it is not always clear and the patient's wishes are not always known. Are they doing what the patient wants? And if it is what the patient wants, is it because he truly understands the impli-cations of his directions? In addition to the intense workloads and complex medical conditions nurses already face, constant worry about whether the care they are giving is really in the patient's best interest can be enough over the long term to turn nurses away from their field, espe-cially in critical care units. (Understandably, as reported earlier, the vacancy rates in intensive care units are higher than other areas of a hos-pital.) To assist the healthcare team and itself, the public needs greater involvement in the debate about when aggressive medical treatment should be stopped and palliative comfort measures begun.

For family members, the moment of crisis is a terrible time to be faced with a decision. Grief, fear, guilt, and desire to do what is right makes such a decision heart wrenching at the very least and leaves a mark that may forever haunt the survivors. Complicating the decisions are the images shown on popular hospital-based television shows. A patient who is wheeled into the emergency room with an emergency medical technician pushing on his chest and another squeezing a bag to help give him oxygen is more often than not revived. (In 1996, researchers reported that patients on television hospital shows survived 75 percent of the time following CPR in the field.)[1] The implication is that the patient eventually leaves the hospital under his own power with his mental faculties intact. In real life the outcome is much more grim. Few good statistics exist about the success of CPR that is started "in the field," or away from the hospital, but reports have been anywhere from a dismal 0 percent to an optimistic 20 percent.[2] And neurological damage resulting from the brain being deprived of oxygen is not factored in. It is estimated that within two to four minutes after the heart has stopped beating, brain damage can begin.

In 1991 the Patient Self-Determination Act (PSDA) was passed, requiring all hospitals and healthcare organizations that receive Medicare and Medicaid to provide patients with written material that states that they have the right to accept or refuse medical or surgical treatment. When adult patients are admitted to the hospital, they are asked if they have any written directive and must be alerted to the fact that they may file a complaint if their provider of care does not comply with their wishes. Healthcare organizations are also required to provide education about advance directives to their staff and the community. The Joint Commission on Accreditation of Healthcare Organizations has included advance directive regulations in its survey process, and the American Medical Association and the American Nurses Association have both included advance care components as part of their professional practice recommendations.

The PSDA arose from some famous cases in which family members were at odds with the healthcare organizations about what actions should be taken to sustain life. Ethical questions arose about the conflict between what can be done and what should be done. In 1976 California was the first state to pass a law that gave patients and those they designate the right to refuse treatment that would sustain life. The law carried with it many restrictions, but it did open the way for other court cases and legislation that followed, culminating in the PSDA of 1991. Though more than a decade has passed, however, only 25 percent of Americans currently have some kind of advance directive.[3]

There are many barriers to advance planning, on the side of both the healthcare consumer and the medical field. It is a difficult subject to broach for many people. Understanding the elements involved in end-of-life care requires that most people speak to their physician, and during ever-shorter office visits there may be little time. Physicians are also often reluctant to bring up the subject for a variety of reasons. They may fear that the discussion itself will communicate to their patients that death is imminent. Then again, they may believe that advance directives are not really useful, that patients don't have the ability to understand treatment decisions,[4] or it could simply be that death is an uncomfortable subject for the physician.

But with the gray areas that have evolved around the definitions of life and death, it becomes increasingly important that each person understands and decides how she feels about death and extending life in various situations. The choice about when life-sustaining activities should be initiated or continued and when they should not clearly needs to belong to the individual. Even the family physician cannot always be trusted with such a choice, because the doctor's choice may reflect his own rather than his patient's values.

In Mike Berry's case, the doctor was able to state clearly what his status was. This was helpful to his wife, but she was still faced with a horrible choice. Rather than choose, she delayed. Mike was moved to the intensive care unit, where he spent seventy-two hours while the family gathered and discussed their alternatives. In his little room in the ICU, he was surrounded by equipment and monitors. A tube was down his throat, IV lines hung like vines, and wires were attached to his chest. The family could visit for only short periods while nurses hovered in attendance. Mike's wife and two sons finally agreed that he wouldn't want to continue in that condition and asked that he be removed from the ventilator.

For the family it was a poor experience, leaving them not only with guilt, but with a final picture of Mike surrounded by tubes and instruments, which was so unlike the vital man he had been. For the nurses, it was equally discouraging. It felt like an exercise in futility. They monitored him vigilantly, but with the constant question in their minds of why they were forstalling certain death. The final insult came for the widow in the form of the hospital bill. Tremendous amounts of resources were spent trying to revive Mike in his final hours, and the bill showed it.

(Most insurance pays only 80 percent of charges, leaving the patient and/or the family with the remaining 20 percent.) For the widow, the high cost of caring for her deceased husband must have seemed like a cruel irony.

Hilda Sanford's story was a little different. Since her hip replacement was a voluntary surgery and scheduled in advance, the hospital had sent her an admission packet that included a copy of a sample advance directive. In it, her rights as a patient were explained and terms were defined. Sample questions and answers were offered in language that she could understand and at the end was a form for her to complete. She filled out the form and gave one to her husband and one to the hospital. On her form, she checked that she chose no written guidelines but had directed her agent (in this case, her husband) to make decisions based on her known values. When Mr. Sanford arrived on the scene as the resuscitation team was working frantically to revive his wife, the doctor explained what they were doing and her status. She was so young, he was reluctant to give up, but when Mr. Sanford asked if she would be likely to walk out of the hospital with her mental faculties intact, the doctor acknowledged that even if the team was able to get her heart back to a normal rhythm, there was no telling how long her brain had been deprived of oxygen. She was unlikely to survive without significant neurological damage. As painful as it was, the choice was clear for Mr. Sanford. Hilda had told him she wanted to live more than anything, but only if she could participate in her usual everyday activities and hold and love her new grandbaby. Mr. Sanford asked the team to stop CPR.

The issue of advance directives for patients who have long-term chronic diseases, while even more essential, is sometimes less clear. Often their dying is the end of a long process and the changes are not so significant as for Mike and Hilda, otherwise healthy people who were suddenly struck down. For the chronically ill, death comes in increments. They may have had multiple hospitalizations over an extended period of time, each time inching toward increased disability. They often need guidance in making decisions about their continued care, in deciding at what point they have crossed the line and want to switch from curative to palliative (comfort only) care. And because of the nature of disease, a patient with a chronic illness may find that her line may vary from day to day. Fortunately, the nature of advance directives is that they can be as fluid as the patient wishes them to be. At any time, they can be revised to reflect the patient's desire.

A friend told me about the death of her father, a man in complete control of his faculties, who entered the hospital for back surgery. Complications ensued and a whole cascade of events followed over a period of several months, during which time he was unable to leave the hospital. Prior to his admission, they had discussed his advance directives. He strongly stated that if heroic measures were required to save his life and the outcome meant spending the remainder of his life in a wheelchair, he did not want to be resuscitated. However, as the months passed and the complications resulting from his back surgery left him confined to his bed, the discussions continued. His line began to move. Losses that had previously seemed unacceptable were reconsidered. Remaining in a wheelchair was no longer deemed unmanageable compared to the alternative. Fortunately, with open communication both the daughter and the hospital were able to stay up-to-date with his changing feelings and when the time ultimately came, his daughter, as his agent for medical decisions, was able to make hers based on an understanding of what he desired. It is easy to see how different the experience might have been for all involved, including the nurses who cared for him over several months, had father and daughter not repeatedly discussed his wishes.

Several groups are working together to promote better end-of-life care and to help people make informed decisions about the care they desire. Last Acts, a national coalition whose goal is to improve care and caring near the end of life, publishes on its Web site a list of important legal issues that people should understand when planning end-of-life care:

1. A competent person has the right to be free of unwanted medical treatment even if the result is death. And if they cannot communicate, all fifty states have procedures for how those decisions will be made.

2. Advance directives are legal documents. They can either give directions about desired care or appoint someone as a proxy. Each state has its own rules.

3. The Patient Self-Determination Act is a federal law requiring that healthcare organizations inform patients of their rights concerning advance directives.

4. Do-Not-Resuscitate (DNR) orders are used in hospitals and can only be assigned by a doctor. It instructs other healthcare providers not to do CPR in the case of cardiac or respiratory arrest.

5. Advance directives will not be followed in emergencies if 911 is called, but many states now allow for a nonhospital DNR order signed by a physician that can be honored by emergency personnel. A DNR is not a do-not-treat order, but only applies to resuscitation.

6. Tube feeding is a medical treatment and a form of life support, but state laws vary about removing it when patients are unable to communicate.

7. Physician-assisted suicide is legal only in Oregon and only under certain conditions. It is defined as a physician knowingly prescribing a lethal dose of drugs for a terminally ill patient to self-administer.

8. Euthanasia is not legal in any state. It involves directly causing death to relieve suffering.

9. Giving drugs for pain that have the unintended consequence of shortening life is not euthanasia.

10. Withholding or withdrawing unwanted medical treatment is not euthanasia. However, state laws may dictate how it can be done.

11. Brain death refers to the irreversible loss of all brain function, and most states legally define death to include brain death. A person in a vegetative state where there is not a loss of all brain function is not officially and legally "brain dead," so life support may be continued.[5]

Last Acts comprises more than one thousand partner organizations and is funded by the Robert Wood Johnson Foundation. The coalition produced a report card for the nation on the availability of services for the dying entitled "Means to a Better End: A Report on Dying in America Today," which gave dismal grades to nearly every state for their relative lack of services. Their findings noted that 28 percent of Medicare patients were admitted to an ICU where aggressive care was given during the last six months of life, often at the expense of comfort; that although 70 percent of Americans state that they would prefer to die at home, only 25 percent did; that many states tied the hands of physicians to keep them from prescribing appropriate pain medication doses for the dying; and that although hospice care is the gold standard, it is not widely used. The report also indicated that few healthcare professionals were trained in palliative care.

Last Acts also released the results of a public opinion poll indicating that the majority of Americans are critical of the care received by the dying in this country. Three-quarters of those surveyed rated the healthcare system as fair or lower on assuring that families' savings were not depleted by end-of-life care. And half indicated that hospitals did only a fair or poor job of providing spiritual or emotional support for the dying.

In a survey of nurses and doctors about the care of patients at the end of life, nearly half reported that they acted against their conscience in providing care for these patients and four times as many were concerned that they had overtreated rather than undertreated.[6] For the nurse, it becomes more difficult because while the doctor may be prescribing a treatment, it is the nurse who is left to carry it out. One oncology nurse explained it this way: "Doctors may want to push on. The nurses know that the patients don't want to continue, that they're ready to go, but if the patients haven't clearly communicated their desires, nurses are caught in the middle."

Who should talk to patients about advance directives remains an issue not clearly defined. Many physicians feel it is their exclusive domain, but not all nurses agree. As the primary caretakers, nurses often feel that they are closer to the patient and the family and are better able to sense when the patient is ready to move to comfort rather than active treatment measures.

The debate about who should address advance directives with

patients is just one of the barriers to supportive end-of-life care erected by the healthcare system. Certainly advances in medicine encourage institutions to take a more aggressive approach to cure, with an increasing focus on prolonging life to the extent permitted by available technology. At the same time, public expectations have risen. Even for those who are elderly, there is often a perception that still more can and should be done. The increasing number of illnesses that have become chronic rather than terminal have also hindered the process. With long-term chronic disease, patients often face one crisis after another. When they are continually pulled back from the brink of death, expectations can increase on the part of both the patient and the physician that it can—and should—be done again.

Though it is recommended that people with long-term illnesses consider hospice benefits within the six-month window prior to death, it rarely happens. Often people are not referred to hospice care until within a few days or weeks of their death, depriving them of the opportunity to avail themselves of the holistic, palliative services offered. I asked a hospice nurse why she thought this happened, and she told of a conversation she had had with a physician. He told her of caring for patients with chronic illnesses, saying that sometimes those relationships spanned a ten- to fifteen-year period, during which time he became increasingly emotionally invested. The number of crises they faced together made it difficult for him to discern when the patient's quality of life had significantly deteriorated, so that sometimes the conversation about changing from aggressive to palliative care came too late. In the face of chronic illness it is all the more imperative to begin discussions of the patient's definition of good end-of-life care while the illness is in its earliest stages.

A young woman told of attending the funeral of an even younger accident victim. She said the shock of it made her and her husband recognize the possibility of their own deaths, and they began discussing what type of funeral and burial they would prefer. Though it was a sobering conversation, they ultimately felt some relief knowing that their wishes had been voiced. And that is the goal of an advance directive: to communicate personal beliefs and wishes well before the need for difficult decisions arises.

Just as with taking responsibility for the effects of lifestyle on one's health, participating in discussions about advance directives is one way that the public can positively affect the nursing shortage. Communicating their desires will not only help nurses in critical care areas avoid the feelings of burnout that are common among them, but the public's understanding of what is meant by aggressive and palliative care will very likely reduce the amount of aggressive care that is given in the final days of life and therefore reduce some of the pressure on already overtaxed resources.

NOTES

1. Stefan Timmermans, *Sudden Death and the Myth of CPR* (Philadelphia: Temple University Press, 1999), p. 84.

2. Ibid., p. 83.

3. Joyce Bedoian, "Did This Patient Die Twice?" *American Journal of Bioethics* [online], http://bioethics.net/inc_er.php?task=view&articleID=690 [October 04, 2002].

4. Bernard J. Hammes and Linda Briggs, *Respecting Choices: Advance Care Planning* (LaCrosse, Wis.: Gunderson Lutheran Medical Foundation, 2000).

5. "Decision Making Isn't Just a Family Matter," Last Acts [online], www.lastacts.org [2001].

6. Karin T. Kirchhoff et al., "End-of-Life Care: Intensive Care Nurses' Experiences with End-of-Life Care," *American Journal of Critical Care* 9, no.1 (January 2000).

CHAPTER ELEVEN
Liability and Healthcare

I n interviews, some nurses have described the chilling effect of liability issues on the workplace. For a few it is the final insult in an
already difficult environment, enough to turn them away from the
field. For nurses trying to do their best each day to help people, finding
themselves named in a lawsuit can be particularly discouraging.

NAMING NURSES

Nurses are not the usual targets of lawsuits as they do not have deep
pockets; they rarely possess enough wealth to warrant the effort; and, as
employees, they generally fall under the hospital's liability coverage.
However, they are often individually named as an agent of the hospital.
One nurse told me of the shock of finding her name on a subpoena.
The case involved a patient of whom she had no recollection, and the
incident for which he was suing had taken place nearly two years earlier. Even after reading the record, she had no memory of caring for him
and was therefore unable to defend herself. Though her name was ultimately dropped from the suit, she said it changed the way she looked
at patients. Where she once felt open, she now feels suspicious and
finds herself monitoring her every word.

Other nurses echoed her sentiment, saying that a patient who wants to write everything down used to be seen as harmlessly if overly cautious. Now if a nurse walks into a room and notes that every action he takes and every word he speaks is being recorded in some fashion, he immediately presumes a lawsuit is imminent.

THE EFFECTS OF LITIGATION

The study by the Institute of Medicine reported in earlier chapters indicates that medical errors are certainly occurring, some of which have grave consequences for patients. Sometimes they result in death or the removal of a healthy limb; other times it may be as simple as giving a medication later than ordered. Even though the complexity of modern healthcare may have increased the number of possible errors, the sheer number of lawsuits and the amount of the monetary settlements awarded also exact an enormous toll on the entire healthcare system.

In Charleston, West Virginia, surgeons conducted a walkout in January 2003 to protest the cost of their medical malpractice insurance rates, while demanding that the state government take action. In Pennsylvania a similar walkout was averted when the governor stepped in with promises of aid, while in Texas legislation to cap malpractice awards was already being considered. New Jersey physicians were protesting by closing their offices. *Forbes* magazine reported that the average jury award for medical malpractice cases tripled between 1994 and 2002, to $3.5 million dollars.[1] Some physicians report that their insurance costs have more than outstripped their ability to earn an income. In Las Vegas one obstetrician said he was closing his practice as his malpractice insurance jumped from $33,000 to $108,000 a year. A Philadelphia orthopedist moved to another state when his malpractice climbed by $50,000.[2] While the growing medical malpractice rates are felt more painfully by physicians, the increase is also being seen at the hospital level. Television journalist and former judge Catherine Crier asserts that one-quarter of the cost of a tonsillectomy and one-third the cost of a pacemaker are directly attributable to litigation expenses.[3]

More insidious than the direct cost of lawsuits, however, is the indirect cost: the defensive actions taken to avoid their possibility. Expensive tests and extra procedures are often ordered out of fear rather than genuine need. And if that happens only 1 percent of the time, the added financial burden can be significant for insurers and hospitals as well as the patients served.

But for nurses, it is not about the financial impact. For them, lawsuits take a much deeper emotional toll. People tend to join the profession for its intrinsic value, to feel as if they are making a difference in the life of another. For a nurse to be named in a lawsuit, even if it is only due to a scattershot approach by lawyers who simply name every caretaker whose signature appears in the chart, it can feel like a betrayal, a cause for questioning whether all the care she is giving, the weekends and holidays sacrificed, is even valued.

The purpose of medical malpractice lawsuits is to help parties who are harmed through negligence to recoup the cost of damages to their health, as well as lost productivity. They are also intended to help rid a system of incompetent practitioners and modify undesirable or careless behaviors in physicians and nurses. These are the desirable outcomes of litigation against doctors and nurses: compensation for harm that is caused by carelessness. Certainly in healthcare, where the potential for injury to the vulnerable is great, some kind of enforcement system must be in place. The question is whether our current system is the best method of equitably serving both the consumer and the provider. Does it have the desired effect of altering careless or negligent behavior, or does it serve only to inhibit those who are already conscientious?

From my own perspective as a nurse, it appears that one negative outcome of litigation is that it creates adversarial relationships where alliances need to be built—between doctor, nurse, and patient. Trust is an essential ingredient between all members of the healthcare team, including the patient. In a system where litigation is the only means of correcting and compensating for significant errors, it is difficult to establish trust and a genuine sense of a shared goal. The patient, for instance, is frightened into feeling that he must always be vigilant or his doctor or nurse may make a terrible error and not tell him. The doctor or nurse may feel that if an honest error is made—even one that causes no harm—it must be hidden from the patient for fear of a lawsuit. And each has reason to fear. Compounding the issue is that the litigation system is full of imperfections. Though there are many legitimate cases that result in the negligent compensating the victim, there are many cases in which justice is not served. Many are settled by insurance companies simply because it may be less costly to settle than to incur the legal fees of defending the innocent. Some are unfairly won or lost due to the varying litigation talents of the lawyers representing either side rather than the relative merits of the case. And worse, in some instances plaintiffs may never bring legitimate cases to court due to lack of understanding of the judicial system.

Clearly the number of cases and the amount of awards have risen in the last decade. Some of that could be attributed to increasing errors in an increasingly complicated medical environment, but it may be beneficial to look at other factors that precipitate a lawsuit and consider which of those can be appropriately controlled.

THE MANAGEMENT OF EXPECTATIONS

Over the last ten years, I have had the opportunity to review a number of potential medical malpractice situations and offer my opinion on the relative liability of a hospital and its nurses. There were instances in which the healthcare provider may have violated the standard of care, but it was not the only reason that lawsuits were initiated. The following are some of the most common reasons I observed: unrealistic patient expectations unmoderated by adequate communication from the physicians managing the case; generalized fear and suspicion; too little time given by doctors and nurses; lack of an adequate system of social supports outside of healthcare; and a pervasive sense that everyone is entitled to compensation for loss.

Some of these factors need to be controlled from within the healthcare system itself. The greatest is the management of expectations. For many reasons, such as the many well-publicized advances that have occurred in healthcare and the increasing longevity of the general population, people have distanced themselves from the truth that humans are still mortal. While it is true that medicine can offer much more than it did thirty, twenty, or even ten years ago, mortality has only been postponed, not "cured." In the last decade, more than once have I heard family members exclaim when speaking of elderly relatives who suddenly died, "How could this have happened? He was so healthy." Grief notwithstanding, a more realistic question might be how he could have lived so well for so long. After reaching a peak of development in early adulthood (younger for some body systems, a little older for others) the human body begins a slow decline. Around age fifty, the immune system starts to lose effectiveness (one reason that 77 percent of all cancers are diagnosed after age fifty-five). At the turn of the century, before antibiotics, the average life span was only around half of today's life expectancy, and even the newest technologies and drugs cannot halt the aging process. They can only delay it. Although good hygiene, healthy habits, and access to medications decrease a person's risk of premature death, all of us must still face our ultimate demise.

To better illustrate, an example can be used of two men entering the hospital for relatively simple appendectomies. One man is twenty-one years of age and the other is seventy-seven. They are facing the same procedure. Both will have general anesthesia and the surgery will take about the same amount of time. Both have an expectation of surviving. However, the older man also faces a higher risk of complications following the surgery. Due to his age, he might be more prone to a blood clot forming in a vein or pneumonia resulting from diminished activity while he recuperates. And if he does suffer one of those complications, he faces a higher risk of his one problem leading to others. The surgeon may understand this, but the patient's and the family's expectations might be that all appendectomies carry the same risk and that a death resulting from complications following surgery must be someone's fault, that is, due to negligence. In the doctor's defense, the extra care required in communication was not always so essential. Twenty years ago, an oncologist could tell her patient that some treatment or medication would help the patient "feel better." Both the patient and the doctor would understand that those words did not mean that what the doctor was prescribing would cure the patient, only that it would ease suffering. Now, patients need to hear very clearly what the expected outcome of a treatment will be in order to avoid misunderstandings. If the family of a patient with long-term chronic obstructive pulmonary disease is told that he needs to be put on a ventilator to help with his breathing, they also need to be told what the chances are that the patient will live to get off the ventilator. They need to hear whether his body needs rest while fighting a lung infection or if he is being put on the ventilator with the expectation that he will die there.

A Culture of Fear

A patient often enters the healthcare system suspicious and fearful about the care she might receive. Some of the fear is generated as a result of studies that demonstrate that real medical errors do occur in hospitals, but those feelings may be compounded by sensationalized media presentations. With twenty-four-hour television news networks and numerous prime-time newsmagazines, it is easy to see how the emotional angles of certain stories can be replayed repeatedly. For instance, in February 2003 a tragic story transpired when a young girl received an organ transplant from a donor who had an incompatible blood type. Her body rejected the transplant and she died after a second transplant surgery failed to correct the problem. This was truly a tragic situation, but the endless coverage received may have done more than inform. It also wrenched at peoples' hearts and inspired fear in those watching. Of all the coverage I observed, I never heard about the number of flawless procedures carried out in the United States or how many lives that particular surgeon had previously saved. Little if any emphasis was put on the fact that without the surgery the young girl's death was not only certain, but imminent. Without putting the story into perspective, the impression left by the media is that everyone is at great risk if they need healthcare. The resulting apprehension helps set the tone for increasing lawsuits, especially when combined with unrealistic expectations of healthcare's capabilities. People who face a negative outcome of their illness or injury are more likely to believe it was someone's fault if they are already fearful.

At the same time law firms are advertising for clients who have been injured by the carelessness of others and claiming that their skills instill fear into the insurance companies and often result in the awarding of huge judgments. Again, it is easy to see how their claims, coupled with the implication that anyone who has suffered deserves compensation, might encourage people toward more lawsuits, especially if the villain is depicted as an anonymous (and believed to be a deep-pocketed) insurance company, hospital, or doctor.

TOO LITTLE TIME

Unfortunately, the increasingly complicated task of caring for people has meant decreased time for doctors and nurses to spend with each patient. The unintended consequence is that patients feel forgotten and uncared for. Ironically it is when the caretakers have the least time that they are most needed, for just as understanding the intricacies of new technology and treatments has become challenging to those inside healthcare, it has also proven bewildering to the public. It can be daunting to try to understand precisely the function of each machine or medicine within a complicated treatment regimen without a medical background. As a result, the patient's and family's understanding may be incomplete. If one nurse or physician does something in one way and another does it in a slightly different way, it may be misinterpreted as an error. Since the patients don't feel particularly well cared for, it may also be interpreted as an intentional slight. To help raise patients' level of understanding requires that nurses and doctors have more time to spend with them, not something that is readily available in our current system.

FALLING THROUGH THE CRACKS

With the publicity of huge monetary awards, people cannot help but privately consider how they can also cash in, especially if they are struggling financially. A hospital chaplain told me of a woman who became ill while also caring for an elderly parent and raising two children alone. With her own illness and its treatment, she became unable to work. Desperate, she sought disability and was told she didn't qualify. She faced the possible loss of her home and an inability to continue to provide for her children and parents. She had worked hard all her life and yet when she was unable, there was no safety net available to her. The woman did not have an attitude of entitlement, and she did not believe that she was "owed" for her hardships, but when pushed to desperate limits, she could be a "lawsuit waiting to happen." In her situation, there was little social assistance available. She was not yet impoverished enough to receive aid, yet if she became that impoverished, she would have a difficult time ever recovering from her losses. In other words, she fell through the cracks. What she wouldn't choose ordinarily she might resort to rather than see her family suffer.

Assigning Blame

Though not true of the woman described above, sometimes a factor in the initiation of a lawsuit is the belief that if something bad happens to someone, the one who is suffering is entitled to compensation. People seek someone to blame for their misfortune. If a complication follows a surgery, the surgeon or the nurse might be blamed. The assumption is natural, but the reasoning can be faulty. Just because a complication follows a surgery doesn't implicate the surgeon. He could have done everything perfectly and a poor outcome occurred in spite of his best efforts. Therefore there is no basis for punishing him.

Necessary Changes

Clearly something is lacking with the system when it is perceived that the only way to right a wrong or to get the financial help needed is through litigation. There need to be other mechanisms in place. It might start with increased self-policing in healthcare. Hospitals have to face the JCAHO surveys and accreditations, and nurses as employees are monitored both by their employers and a fairly rigorous board of nursing. Physicians, however, who place a high value on autonomy, are not known for their willingness to police themselves or others within their profession. A nurse has to conform to the standards of practice or is quickly severed from employment, but physicians have less oversight. A more rigorous effort within the profession to rid itself of those who are not competent might help restore public confidence and reduce the burden of lawsuits for the vast majority who strive to be excellent clinicians.

Another important change that needs to take place is building more time into healthcare. That will require cooperation from many different groups. Insurers have to recognize the amount of time needed by providers and be prepared to increase reimbursement. Time-efficient tools need to be implemented by hospitals to help reduce the paperwork and documentation to allow for more time with patients. And with increased time, more emphasis must be placed on educating the public. Like any specialty group, medicine has its own language and it needs to be carefully interpreted to the patient to help him more fully function as the most important member of his healthcare team.

The system of litigation itself may need an overhaul, something that legislators are currently considering. Caps applied to the noneconomic damages do not limit the amount a patient can fairly be awarded for medical bills incurred or time lost from work as a result of someone's carelessness, but it does stop huge punitive awards.

There could also be a cap applied to the amount a lawyer can earn from one case. Most medical malpractice cases are performed on a contingency basis, with 30 or 40 percent of the award paid to the lawyer if the suit is successful. The benefit of such a system is that anyone who has a claim cannot be prevented from action simply because she lacks the funds to hire a lawyer. At the same time, inherent in such a system is the temptation to sue for more than would reasonably compensate for the loss. A challenge to legislators would be to find alternative means of serving both the patients who have a grievance as well as the healthcare system that needs to answer for its actions. Perhaps panels of medical professionals and laypeople could hear grievances and give awards within a defined scope. All potential cases could be reviewed prior to being entered into the court system and a penalty taken from a lawyer who knowingly initiates a frivolous suit. At the same time, professional organizations can be charged with stricter policing of their own or face significant fines. And, of course, the public has a role, perhaps the most difficult of all in light of our current state. Our challenge is to take responsibility for our health and actively participate in our healthcare—to ask questions when we don't understand; to know the medications we take and the dosages; to remember that there is not always blame to be assigned, not even to ourselves, and that unexplainable things happen that are outside the control of humans. There is a better answer and change doesn't have to wait. It only takes a few strong voices for reason to help point us in a new direction.

NOTES

1. Michael Freedman, "Critical Condition," *Forbes* 169, May 13, 2002, p. 19.

2. Mary Brophy Marcus, "Healthcare's 'Perfect Storm,'" *U.S. News & World Report*, July 1, 2002, p. 39.

3. Catherine Crier, *The Case against Lawyers* (New York: Broadway Books, 2002), p. 14.

CHAPTER TWELVE
Three West Revisited

This is not a story with an unhappy ending. Already forces are at work to change conditions within and beyond nursing that will enhance the working environment for nurses while creating safer environments for patients. And through more collaborative practice, increasingly satisfying working environments will be created for physicians as well. Everyone has the opportunity to benefit. Even the hospitals who will incur the initial costs of creating magnetlike atmospheres will more than recoup their costs in quality of care and reduced turnover of personnel. If at least a few Americans can begin to alter their health habits and curb the rate of preventable chronic diseases, healthcare may be able to remain fiscally sound!

To get an idea of how different nursing looks when everything is working, let's revisit Karen's fateful Saturday as a new charge nurse on Three West.

Karen Hensley stepped off the elevator into the darkened halls of Three West and breathed in the familiar hospital smells. It was 6:30 A.M. She was early, but it was her first day as the shift charge nurse and she wanted time to review the room assignments before the rest of the staff arrived. She liked Saturdays. They were more relaxed than weekdays;

patients had fewer tests and procedures, the operating room was open only to emergencies, and the doctors had time for questions since they didn't have office hours awaiting them. The day had potential. She flipped the light switch and watched the hallway illuminate.

"Good morning," said Carol, the night shift charge nurse. "You're early. Your first day in charge, right? Good, 'cause I need to let you know that Melinda isn't coming in today. The baby's sick. But we called Stacey and she's going to cover, so staffing looks pretty good." She held out the assignment sheet with Stacey's name written above Melinda's.

Karen glanced at the sheet. "Thanks for taking care of that. We would have been short without a replacement. What's our census? We were full when I left Thursday."

"Still are, but most of them are new since then. These short stays are rough. Looks like quite a few discharges planned for today, but you'll probably fill up as soon as they go out the door. Flu season, you know," said Carol.

"Who's the supervisor? Does she know about the switch with Melinda and Stacey?"

Carol nodded. "She said she had some surprise help she was sending you, too, so be on the lookout."

The phone rang and Karen reached for it. "Three West, Karen speaking. How can I help you?"

It was Alice Smart, the nursing supervisor. "Good morning, Karen. Did Carol tell you about your surprise help? Jerry Standhill decided that since he was too busy to get away from the office during the week, he'd come in today and help as a transportation aide."

Karen heard the ding of the elevator and looked up to see Elizabeth, the unit clerk, with Jerry Standhill, the hospital CEO, at her side dressed in scrubs. "Uh, yes, I believe he is here now. What should I do with him?" Karen whispered into the phone.

"He's at your disposal. I'd have him empty the laundry carts, give out water pitchers, that kind of thing. Call me if you need anything."

Rachel and Lilly arrived via the stairs. "Good morning," Lilly called cheerfully, "I'm your mentor today, Karen, so if you have any questions, just ask and I'll try to help."

Karen smiled. "Thanks, I'll need it." The she turned to the CEO,

"Good morning, Mr. Standhill. Nice of you to help us out this morning. Any particular assignment you'd like?"

"Call me Jerry. I pour a mean water pitcher and I hear you've got a number of discharges this morning so I can take the patients downstairs if that will help."

"Hey, who's the cute new guy in the scrubs?" Lilly teased. She and Jerry had started at the hospital on the same day twenty years earlier.

Karen headed to the meeting room to check out the assignments. Twenty-nine patients, three empty beds, six RNs, one LPN, one CNA, plus Jerry—Karen liked the math. The patients would be of a high-intensity level, however. Seven of the patients were unable to feed or bathe themselves and required total care. Five were only one day post-op and would need extra attention and teaching. Three were on isolation precautions requiring that the nurses don gown, mask, and gloves each time they went into the room, and one was beginning the alcohol abuse protocol. He was the wild card. The medications authorized by the protocol could help him sleep through the worst of his withdrawal or he could become frightened and confused, even hostile.

As the other nurses entered for morning report, Karen asked about their assignment preferences. "Shall we all pick or do you just want me to assign?"

Rachel spoke up. "My vote is for you to go ahead and assign. They come and go so fast we don't know them one day to another anyway."

Karen looked at Lilly, who nodded in agreement. "Fine with me."

Karen quickly looked over the roster. Lilly was the most senior staff, and the best. She was a different person than from when Karen had started. She had been so angry then that Karen had been a little afraid of her. But Marie, the unit manager, had assured her that Lilly was just overwhelmed and would feel better once they changed their practice to a team-based approach and improved their staffing ratios. Marie had been right. Lilly had blossomed. She had turned into a dynamo. No challenge was too big for Lilly! Rachel was the novice, but Emma was acting as her preceptor. And Bill and Stacey were experienced RNs who were sharing oversight of Donna's patients since she was an LPN. Then there were Jerry and Robin, the CNA. Karen quickly divided the rooms and asked Robin to assist with the total-care patients.

"Five to one, great ratios for a weekend, don't you think? This is going to be a good day!" said Lilly. "Let's get report started so we can go to work."

Everyone started laughing as Carol began reporting. "I'd better tell you about Mr. Templeton first. He's had a busy night. He's been getting up and wandering. He visited 314 and scared the poor women. I didn't have enough people to assign him a one-on-one, so we brought him out with us. He's in the geriatric chair with the tray. We've gotten him up every hour and walked him around, but he just can't seem to sleep. He needs watching, he said."

Carol completed the remaining patients and then the group broke up. Jerry stayed behind for a minute. "I'll start down the hall with water pitchers, but if you need me, call."

Dr. Felton was waiting for Karen. "I ordered a stat hematocrit yesterday on Mr. Helmsley and the results aren't on the chart. I still haven't figured out the computer system. Can you help me?"

"Be glad to, Dr. Felton. If you have time, I'll show you the keystrokes again."

Elizabeth was standing at the counter where charts with new orders were collecting. She grinned, but made no commentary.

Rachel rushed to the nurses'station. "Quick, is Mr. Turner a DNR? I can't find a pulse."

Emma materialized and led Rachel back to the room, "It's marked on his bracelet, remember? I'll help you check."

Karen grabbed the chart from the rack and skimmed the orders. "He's a DNI (Do Not Intubate)," she called as she headed to the room. "Elizabeth, call a code. Robin, grab the cart."

Feet pounded down the hall as "Code 12" was sounded over the loudspeakers. The room filled with members of the code team even as Rachel and Emma were checking for breath sounds. A back board was pulled from the cart and slid under the patient. CPR was started.

"Who is this? What's the diagnosis? Is he a full code?" asked the ER physician who responded to the code.

"Joseph Turner, admitted yesterday from a nursing home with possible pneumonia. He's a DNI. Rachel found him without a pulse when she was making her morning rounds," Emma explained.

Karen backed out of the door, "I'll call his doctor and see how he wants to proceed."

The ER doctor continued to call orders and a nurse from the code team responded by administering emergency medications through the patient's IV line.

Karen reached the patient's doctor and explained what had happened. He asked to speak with the attending physician. She transferred the call to the room.

"We'll continue for another few minutes," said the physician. "Dr. Hellman wants to call Mr. Turner's son."

"Clear!" a nurse called as she discharged an electrical shock to the man's chest through the paddles.

Five minutes passed before Elizabeth popped her head into the room. "Dr. Hellman is on the line. I'll transfer the call."

After conferring on the phone, the ER doctor ended the code. "Mr. Turner's son is aware of the circumstances. He had talked with his father and said he wouldn't want us to go on more than a couple of minutes. Why don't we get things cleaned up so his son can come and visit him. Time of death is 7:32."

Karen returned to the desk and called the social worker and asked her to come to the unit in case Mr. Turner's family needed some grief counseling.

Charts with new orders were starting to stack the desk as the doctors made morning rounds. "Who's in charge here?" a surgeon growled.

"I am," Karen volunteered. Jerry, hearing the tone from the hallway, entered the nurses' station to stand beside her.

"Good morning, Dr. Beech," he said pleasantly.

"I ordered a dressing change on Mrs. Garrett last night. It's saturated and making a mess of her bed. Get it taken care of and then I want you to find the nurse who should have changed it last night and write her up." The chart slammed down on the desk.

Karen picked it up. "Dr. Beech, I believe it says right here in the progress notes that the nurses changed the dressing twice, the last time at 5:30 this morning."

"Where does it say that?" he asked.

Karen pointed on the page.

"Huh. Thanks," he said and turned away.

Jerry grinned at Karen and went back to water pitcher duty.

"Karen, I need someone to check blood with me," called Donna.

Stacey was right behind her. "No problem. I'll help you."

Lilly entered the nurses' station. "You haven't met Mrs. Bedford, have you? I think she just came in yesterday. She sounds raspy this morning. I think I'll call the nursing home and talk to someone who knows her."

Lilly looked disturbed when she got off the phone. "The nurse at the nursing home said she had developed a fever, but her breathing was fine. Said she helped her to the bathroom yesterday, too, but today it doesn't look like she has the energy to raise her arm. I'd better call Dr. Canfield."

Rachel came to the counter. "Karen, the pharmacy sent the wrong drug on Mr. Gutshell in 306. And they're saying I need some sort of form to get it corrected, but he wants his medication now."

Karen smiled. "Fill out the form and send it to the pharmacy. They will try to be as quick as they can. And tell Mr. Gutshell that you want to do everything possible to ensure his safety."

"Karen, if you need me, I'll be in with Mrs. Bedford. I want to watch her. Dr. Canfield didn't seem concerned enough to me," said Lilly.

"Karen," Elizabeth was calling. "Mr. Turner's son is on the phone. Hey, and I think Mr. Templeton is trying to go traveling."

Jerry came up the hall just as Elizabeth was calling. Mr. Templeton had slid down under the tray that confined him to the chair, so that his chin was on the tray and his gown was no longer covering all of his parts. "Would you like to get up for a few minutes, Mr. Templeton?" Jerry asked. "Maybe you and I could take a little walk."

Together he and Karen removed the tray and helped Mr. Templeton to his feet. "Here's a robe for him," Emma said. "It might add a little more dignity to your stroll."

Karen watched as the two men walked down the hall toward the patient lounge, then said to Elizabeth, "Too bad we can't get him to work every weekend, huh?"

"The garage," they could hear Mr. Templeton saying. "I need to get out to the garage."

"Do you know where you are? You're in the hospital, Mr. Templeton." . . . Jerry's voice trailed off as they moved out of earshot.

Alice appeared at the desk. "How are you doing this morning? Did you remember to call the eye bank on Mr. Turner?" she asked.

"Yes, it's all taken care of. I called the social worker, too. Should I call the chaplain in or wait and see what the family needs? I hate to bring her in if she isn't needed."

Alice nodded, "I would wait and see. He was an older gentleman, right? It might not be unexpected to the family. Any other surprises today? How is Jerry doing?"

Lilly was back. "Alice, I've got a little situation. What do you think? I've got a patient who has come in from the nursing home. Her condition has completely deteriorated in my mind. Oxygen saturation levels are a little down. Vitals are okay, but she's considerably weaker. And the daughter seems to be expecting that her mother is going to be restored to her former health. Completely restored I mean, the way she was six months ago, before her stroke."

Alice asked, "What do you think?"

"I think that the doctor needs to get in here and talk to her and take a look at her mother."

"Good," Alice said. "I agree. Call him and tell him that and if you need help, we'll go further."

A gentleman approached the desk and stood waiting silently. "How can I help you?" Karen asked.

"My father, Mr. Turner."

"Oh yes, Mr. Turner, we're so sorry for your loss. Have you been in to see him?"

"Yes, I just wanted to say I was leaving. The funeral home has been called," he said. There were tears in his eyes.

"Would you like to speak with someone, Mr. Turner, the chaplain or the social worker?"

He looked down at the floor and shook his head. "No, thanks, I think I'll just be getting on. Thank you."

A frightened woman approached the desk. "My husband is breathing too fast. He says his chest hurts. It's just like when he had his heart attack. He needs the doctor now."

Karen called Bill over the call system and directed him to the room stat, while she checked the patient's order sheet for medication for his chest pain. There was nothing. "Bill," she called as he sailed past the nurses'station, "find out if he's had these episodes at home and what they do for them." She dialed the answering service to alert the doctor on call. Bill returned to report the vital signs. "I'm going to get an EKG," he said, "and put some oxygen on him. The doctor will need the results anyway." He took off down the hall. Three minutes without a return phone call and Karen called the answering service again. "We need him stat," she said firmly.

Three more minutes passed. "Emma," Karen called, "can you go and help Bill? Assure the patient and his wife we're doing everything we can."

Karen dialed the ER and asked for someone to come quickly. Within minutes, a flurry of activity surrounded the patient. The ER physician looked at the EKG rhythm strip and said he needed to get downstairs at once. The man was quickly transferred to a stretcher by Jerry and Bill and they raced to the ER with him, while Emma walked behind gently supporting his wife.

Karen took a deep breath and noticed Mr. Templeton from the corner of her eye. In the rush of the moment, he had been forgotten. She intercepted him just as he was about to step into the elevator. Gently, she took his elbow and guided him back toward the nurses' station. "Why don't you come with me, Mr. Templeton? Are you hungry? I've got some snacks for you in the kitchen."

His head bobbed and he mumbled, "Garage. Just need to get to my garage."

Dr. Canfield appeared at the desk and Lilly came to meet him. She filled him in on Mrs. Bedford and her daughter. "She's never talked to her mother about advance directives. She needs you to help her understand her mother's real condition. She's thinking she's going to start talking again any day now. I called for a bed in ICU just in case you decide to move her."

He frowned. "Do you really think that will be necessary?"

"I don't think it would be Mrs. Bedford's choice, but I bet she can't go on much longer without some help breathing, either," said Lilly.

Together they walked toward Mrs. Bedford's room.

Noon came and went. Jerry ordered a pizza and the nurses and aides grabbed slices on the run.

The patient being discharged from 312 said his dentures were lost, which started a frantic search of his room until a family member acknowledged taking them home for safe keeping.

The nursing supervisor called to say that the evening shift was short and that she was offering incentive pay to anyone willing to work overtime.

Emma walked past the desk with Mr. Paulson. "We're out for our morning walk," she said to Karen. "Now that Mr. Paulson understands how important it is to take care of his diabetes, he's going to start exercising twice a day, just short walks at first, because he has to be careful of his toe, but as soon as that's resolved . . ."

"I'm going to start jogging," Mr. Paulson joked.

Call bells chimed. Intravenous pumps alarmed. The ER called report on the patient with the chest pain and said he was being transferred to ICU. They said the quick action had saved the man's life. Karen made a mental note to tell Bill. Doctors left new orders. Patients were discharged. A weary Dr. Canfield finally returned to the nurses' station and wrote a DNR order on Mrs. Bedford's chart.

Karen raised her eyebrows in question. "Lilly was right," Dr. Canfield said. "She has pneumonia, and from her X ray I'd say it moved really fast. It took a long time to explain to the daughter. She really did still believe her mother was just going to go back to the way she used to be. This is going to really be hard for her. You might ask her if she wants the chaplain."

Karen nodded and patted his shoulder. "How about you? Are you okay?"

"I'll be okay. I'll go home and play with the kids and get some perspective," he said, but he looked very sad as he turned away.

Karen put in the call to the chaplain, who promised to come as soon as she could. Then she went to check on Mrs. Bedford's daughter herself. Lilly was there. They were sitting next to the bed, talking softly. Karen backed out quietly without disturbing them. She passed Bill in the hall. "Great save, Bill," she congratulated him. "The ER said your patient was going to the ICU and he might not have made it if you hadn't moved him out so quickly."

Bill thanked her and chased after Jerry to thank him for his help.

Just as the evening shift was preparing to go into report, Mr. Paulson's daughter approached the desk with a basket of fruit. "Dad asked me to give this to you. Usually he asks me to bring cookies, but he says after all the preaching he's been hearing about health, that you might like fruit better."

Karen started to laugh. "We love fruit. And your dad's doing great, isn't he?"

She nodded. "Yes, the doctor says he'll still have to take the toe, but he said the circulation in the rest of his foot looks good. And now with his new interest in exercise, who knows?" She smiled and continued down the hall.

Karen straightened her shoulders and walked back to the conference room with the fruit basket. She set it on the table. "This is from Mr. Paulson. His daughter said she usually brings cookies—" Karen's voice broke.

"Hey, Karen, don't you like fruit?" The other nurses started to laugh.

Karen continued, "She said he said he's going to change his ways thanks to us."

A hand reached up and ripped at the wrapping. "It's nice when you win some of them, huh?"

Jerry caught up with Karen in the parking lot later. "Jerry," she said when he tapped her shoulder, "you were such a great help. Thanks so much."

Jerry smiled. "You know, that's not fair. You beat me to it. I was coming to thank you. I don't know how you do it everyday, but I'm glad you do."

"Me, too." Karen said and smiled.

After the introduction of self-governance and optimal nurse-to-patient ratios, the Three West nursing unit is a much safer and satisfying place for both the nurses and the patients for whom they care. It doesn't alter the basic fact that people get sick, that some die as a result, and that nursing is often both physically and emotionally challenging. But it does ease the burden by allowing time for the surveillance, health teaching, and emotional support that are essential to good care.

The lack of nurses isn't just a problem confined to the profession, but one that impacts all elements of society. There are few people who can escape the need for nursing care at some point in their lives, which makes it all the more imperative that a nurse's work is valued and that the daily tasks are not so overwhelming as to bury the intrinsic rewards. Each person deserves the kind of care that can be received from dedicated men and women who enter a nurturing vocation by choice. With increasing wages, improving working conditions, exciting technological advances, and the inherent satisfaction of helping others, nursing can once again become the kind of profession parents encourage their children to pursue.

APPENDIX A
Nursing Organizations

GENERAL NURSING ASSOCIATIONS

American Nurses Association
600 Maryland Avenue, SW, Suite 100 West
Washington, DC 20024
800-274-4262
www.ana.org

Canadian Nurses Association
50 Driveway
Ottawa, ON K2P 1E2
Canada
613-237-2133
www.cna-nurses.ca

National Federation of Licensed Practical Nurses, Inc.
605 Poole Drive
Garner, NC 27529
919-779-0046
www.nflpn.org

NURSING LEADERSHIP ASSOCIATIONS

American Organization of Nurse Executives
Liberty Place
325 Seventh Street, NW
Washington, DC 20004
202-626-2240
www.aone.org

National Association of Directors of Nursing Administration
    in Long-Term Care
10101 Alliance Road, #140
Cincinnati, OH 45242
513-791-3679
www.nadona.org

NURSING EDUCATION ORGANIZATIONS AND STATE BOARDS

American Association of Colleges of Nursing
One Dupont Circle, NW, Suite 530
Washington, DC 20036
202-463-6930
www.aacn.nche.edu

National Council of State Boards of Nursing, Inc.
111 East Wacker Drive, Suite 2900
Chicago, IL 60601
312-525-3600
www.ncsbn.org

National League for Nursing
61 Broadway
New York, NY 10006
800-669-1656
www.nln.org

MINORITY NURSING ASSOCIATIONS

American Assembly for Men in Nursing
11 Cornell Road
Latham, NY 12110-1499
518-782-9400, ext. 346
www.aamn.org

National Association of Hispanic Nurses
1501 Sixteenth Street, NW
Washington, DC 20036
202-387-2477
www.thehispanicnurses.org

National Black Nurses Association, Inc.
8630 Fenton Street, Suite 330
Silver Spring, MD 20910-3803
301-589-3200
www.nbna.org

APPENDIX B

Specialty Nursing Organizations

S pecialty nursing organizations are important to the profession. They serve to promote expertise within a specialized area of nursing by promoting research and education, and defining best practices. They offer educational conferences, journals, and opportunities to share knowledge with other nurses with similar interests. Certification exams are available through many specialty organizations, offering nurses the opportunity to earn nationally recognized certifications that demonstrate their specialized knowledge and expertise.

Air & Surface Transport Nurses Association
9101 East Kenyon Avenue, Suite 3000
Denver, CO 80237
800-897-6362
www.astna.org

Academy of Medical-Surgical Nurses
East Holly Avenue, Box 56
Pitman, NJ 08071-0056
856-256-2323
www.medsurgnurse.org

American Academy of Ambulatory Care Nursing
East Holly Avenue, Box 56
Pitman, NJ 08071-0056
856-256-2350
www.aaacn.org

American Association of Critical Care Nurses
101 Columbia
Aliso Viejo, CA 92656-4109
800-899-2226
www.aacn.org

American Association of Diabetes Educators
100 West Monroe Street, Suite 400
Chicago, Illinois 60603
800-338-3633
www.aadenet.org

American Association of Legal Nurse Consultants
401 North Michigan Avenue
Chicago, IL 60611
877-402-2562
www.aalnc.org

American Association of Neuroscience Nurses
4700 West Lake Avenue
Glenview, IL 60025
888-557-2266
www.aann.org

American Association of Nurse Anesthetists
222 South Prospect Avenue
Park Ridge, IL 60068-4001
847-692-7050
www.aana.com

American Association of Occupational Health Nurses, Inc.
2920 Brandywine Road, Suite 100
Atlanta, GA 30341
770-455-7757
www.aaohn.org

American Association of Office Nurses
109 Kinderkamack Road
Montvale, NJ 07645
800-457-7504
www.aaon.org

American Association of Spinal Cord Injury Nurses
75-20 Astoria Boulevard
Jackson Heights, NY 11370
718-803-3782
www.aascin.org

American Board for Occupational Health Nurses, Inc.
201 East Ogden Road, Suite 114
Hinsdale, IL 60521-3652
888–842-2646
www.abohn.org

American College of Cardiovascular Nursing
P.O. Box 61606
Virginia Beach, VA 23466
757-497-4143
www.accn.net

American Forensic Nurses
255 North El Cielo, Suite 195
Palm Springs, CA 92262
760-322-9925
www.amrn.com

American Nephrology Nurses' Association
East Holly Avenue, Box 56
Pitman, NJ 08071-0056
888-600-2662
www.annanurse.org

American Nursing Informatics Association
PMB 105
10808 Foothill Boulevard, Suite 160
Rancho Cucamonga, CA 91730
www.ania.org

American Psychiatric Nurses Association
1555 Wilson Boulevard, Suite 515
Arlington, VA 22209
703-243-2443
www.apna.org

American Radiological Nurses Association
7794 Grow Drive
Pensacola, FL 32514
866-486-2762
www.arna.net

American Society of Pain Management Nursing
7794 Grow Drive
Pensacola, FL 32514
888-342-7766
www.aspmn.org

American Society of Plastic Surgical Nurses
P.O. Box 56
Pitman, NJ 08071-0056
856-256-2340
www.aspsn.org

Association of Perioperative Registered Nurses, Inc.
2170 South Parker Road, Suite 300
Denver, CO 80231
800-755-2676
www.aorn.org

Association of Pediatric Oncology Nurses
4700 West Lake Avenue
Glenview, IL 60025
847-375-4724
www.apon.org

Association of Rehabilitation Nurses
4700 West Lake Avenue
Glenview, IL 60025
800-229-7530
www.rehabnurse.org

Emergency Nurses Association
915 Lee Street
Des Plaines, IL 60016-6569
800-900-9659
www.ena.org

Hospice and Palliative Nurses Association
Penn Center West One, Suite 229
Pittsburgh, PA 15276
412-787-9301
www.hpna.org

Infusion Nurses Society
220 Norwood Park South
Norwood, MA 02062
781-440-9408
www.ins1.org

League of Intravenous Therapy Education
Empire Building, Suite 3
3001 Jacks Run Road
White Oak, PA 15131
412-678-5025
www.lite.org

National Association for Home Care and Hospice
228 Seventh Street, SE
Washington, DC 20003
202-547-7424
www.nahc.org

National Association of Neonatal Nurses
4700 West Lake Ave
Glenview, IL 60025-1485
847-375-3660
www.nann.org

National Association of Pediatric Nurse Practitioners
20 Brace Road, Suite 200
Cherry Hill, NJ 08034-2633
856-857-9700
www.napnap.org

Oncology Nursing Society
125 Enterprise Drive
Pittsburgh, PA 15275-1214
866 257-4667
www.ons.org

Rural Nurse Organization
Letterman Lanning
P.O. Box 248
Spokane, WA 99210-0248
800-752-4890
www.rno.org

Society of Gastroenterology Nurses and Associates, Inc.
401 North Michigan Avenue
Chicago, IL 60611-4267
800-245-7462
www.sgna.org

Society of Trauma Nurses
PMB 300 223 North Guadalupe
Santa Fe, NM 87501
505-983-4923
www.traumanursesoc.org

Society of Urologic Nurses and Associates
East Holly Avenue, Box 56
Pitman, NJ 08071-0056
888-827-7862
www.suna.org

APPENDIX C

Groups Supporting Nurses

American Hospital Association
One North Franklin
Chicago, IL 60606-3421
312-422-3000
www.aha.org

The AHA released a report in May 2002 on the recruitment and retention of nurses: *In Our Hands: Helping Hospital Leaders Build a Thriving Workforce.*

Institute for Safe Medication Practices
1800 Byberry Road, Suite 810
Huntingdon Valley, PA 19006
215-947-7797
www.ismp.org

The ISMP in a nonprofit organization that provides education to healthcare institutions about adverse drug events and their prevention. It offers free educational presentations to nurses as well as a free newsletter.

John A. Hartford Foundation
55 East 59th Street, 16th Floor
New York, NY 10022-1178
212-832-7788
www.jhartfound.org

In support of geriatric nursing, the John A. Hartford Foundation's Building Academic Geriatric Nursing Capacity scholar program selected twenty new nurse scholars to receive up to $100,000 each to support their studies. More information about the program can be found at http://nursingworld.org/aan/news or www.geriatricnursing.org.

Johnson & Johnson Health Care Systems, Inc.
Piscataway, NJ 08855-6800
www.discovernursing.com

Johnson & Johnson committed more than a million dollars in funding for a media campaign to recruit new nurses. Besides television ads, the company launched a comprehensive Web site about nursing with information on required education, and nursing associations, nursing publications, as well as a listing with links to 1,450 nursing programs.

Joint Commission on Accreditation of Healthcare
    Organizations
601 Thirteenth Street, NW, Suite 1150N
Washington, DC 20005
202-783-6655
www.jcaho.org

In August 2002 the JCAHO released a report on the nursing shortage with suggestions for change, entitled "Health Care at the Crossroads."

Josiah Macy Jr. Foundation
44 East 64th Street
New York, NY 10021
212-486-2424
www.josiahmacyfoundation.org

The Josiah Macy Jr. Foundation recently awarded a grant to a project that would provide academic nursing with a faster track so that nurses could reach a PhD level sooner and have more time left to serve as educators.

Robert Wood Johnson Foundation
P. O. Box 2316
College Road East and Route 1
Princeton, NJ 08543
888-631-9989
www.rwjf.org

The Robert Wood Johnson Foundation seeks to improve the health and healthcare of all Americans. It supports training, education, and research. It recently supported a study on the American nursing shortage (see Web site for details).

VHA, Inc.
220 East Las Colinas Boulevard
Irving, TX 75039-5500
www.vha.com

The VHA released the study "The Business Case for Work Force Stability" in November 2002.

W. K. Kellogg Foundation
One Michigan Avenue East
Battle Creek, MI 49017
269-968-1611
www.wkkf.org

The W. K. Kellogg Foundation is a nonprofit organization whose mission is to apply knowledge to solve the problems of people. It recently began the Graduate Medical and Nursing Education Initiative to develop multidisciplinary approaches to the education of medical and nursing specialists. Information can be found at the Web site.

APPENDIX D

Help with Advance Directives

Where can people find help with advance directives? A number of organizations and Web sites offer information about advance directives, including Last Acts (www.lastacts.org). For information about palliative care, the National Hospice and Palliative Care Organization, located in Alexandria, Virginia, has a Web site at www.nhpco.org. The Hospice Foundation of America can be found at www.hospicefoundation.org.

Hospice care is available in many areas of the country and appropriate organizations can usually be found in local telephone listings. Many hospitals also offer regular education programs about advance directives and have written materials that can be a starting point for discussion. Especially important is gaining an understanding of the terms used when speaking of prolonging life, such as intubation. Discussing choices with family and a personal physician ahead of time will later make those decisions much easier.

It is important to remember that end-of-life-care planning isn't just about the moment of death, but also considers the point at which one might choose to discontinue aggressive treatment. Physicians are trained to treat. Until instructed otherwise, they continue to take life-prolonging action. Communicating ahead of time through advance directives allows each person to consider his options while he is cognizant. Whether an individual chooses to have everything done that is possible or chooses to withdraw life-prolonging treatment at a certain point, the goal of advance directives is to ensure that the choice is fully communicated and that individual wishes are followed. Early discussion also allows people to discover the philosophy of their physicians and gives them the opportunity to choose a caregiver whose values reflect their own.

APPENDIX E

Fighting Obesity and Overweight

S tarting at the grade-school level, children should have the opportunity to understand the connection between their actions (or
inactions) and their health. According to some experts, 20 to 30 percent
of children in the United States are overweight, leading to a potentially
significant rate of diabetes in just a few years[1] if nothing is done. High
cholesterol and high blood pressure are also being seen in overweight
children and adolescents,[2] putting them at high risk for heart disease.
But the most immediate consequence for overweight, as perceived by
the children, is social discrimination.[3] Since adults are at least equally
responsible for children's weight, they also need to be educated about
the risks their children face as well as the emotional price they pay. A
weight loss of only 5 to 7 percent coupled with exercise can reduce an
overweight person's risk of diabetes by 58 percent.[4]

For children, exercise is critical and very effective at burning off
extra calories, but a difficult habit to develop when electronics compete
for their attention, especially if their parents are not active. Parents may
need to not only join them, but find a way to make it fun. Physical education programs that have been minimized or cut in many schools have
to regain prominence to ward off the obesity epidemic.

A quick search on the Internet for references to obesity yielded 1.4
million matches. For weight loss, 8,010 sites were given. Obviously,

people are neither unaware of nor unconcerned about the problem. The difficulty is in getting to the "a-ha" moment that will initiate action. Tommy Thompson had his. He announced that while trying to help persuade Americans that they needed to change their lifestyle, he changed his own. He dropped from 215 pounds to 197, working toward his personal goal of 185 pounds.

Oprah Winfrey told the story of her "a-ha" moment, of being at the Emmy Awards and wishing that she wouldn't win so no one would see how broad she had become. In truth, few were judging her weight. Her accomplishments and the adoration of her audiences are legendary, but that didn't change her judgment of herself. And that night, when she should have been feeling incredibly proud, she instead felt shame. Rather than despair, Ms. Winfrey took that dreadful moment and turned it into a great motivator. She was so successful, she went on to run the Marine Corps Marathon in Washington, D.C.—26.3 miles!

Other "a-ha" moments? A guess at Tommy Thompson's would be that he realized the danger of America continuing on its reckless course toward obesity and was preparing to "rally the troops" when he noticed his own girth. Telling others to "do as I say and not as I do" is less effective than leading by example, so he took the lead.

Other "a-ha" moments shared—the moment when the decision was made and resolve was born:

- A daughter's engagement meant the mother of the bride needed a new dress.
- A birthday ending in zero.
- An impending class reunion and the desire to make an old flame feel a little stir.
- Walking one flight of stairs and getting out of breath.
- The birth of a grandchild.
- A blood pressure scare.
- A breast cancer scare.

As for myself, I've had many. I ran the Marine Corps Marathon the same year as Oprah Winfrey, but although I've continued to exercise and—based on blood work—have a relatively low risk of heart disease due to fitness, the research for this chapter frightened me. As a nurse, I have seen the reality. Extra weight creates extra work for every body system, and the parts simply wear out faster. I calculated my own BMI along with Tommy Thompson's, and like him, am wavering on the cusp. I have an only child who has yet to marry, produce children, and win her Oscar. I would hate to leave before the show is over.

What do you do if that moment has arrived? First, make a visit to the family doctor for a general checkup, advice on how much of a weight loss is desirable, and clearance to begin an exercise program. The doctor may also know from other patients' experiences which approaches are most likely to yield success. One task recommended by many weight loss groups is journaling—keeping an accurate account of every bite of food consumed each day, because most people underestimate their intake. Often the awareness that goes with writing it down has an immediate positive effect. Although losing weight is not easy, for the more fortunate, awareness coupled with support from loved ones or from weight loss groups who are working toward a common goal can have a powerful effect. Others may need more assistance.

As a nurse who switched from running up and down halls all day to a desk job, I found that when I stopped moving, I quickly spread to fill the chair. After conferring with various friends, I decided to visit a nutritionist. She asked me to observe my eating patterns and, without trying to change behaviors, to write down what I ate. I complied. Three days later I returned with journal in hand. She read it over carefully without comment. Then she pulled out a calculator and wrote down some figures. The problem, she announced, was that my eating was perfectly reasonable up until 7:00 P.M., at which point all bets were off. I nodded in agreement. So, she continued sagely, I needed to stop eating after seven. I looked her over carefully. Since she appeared to weigh all of one hundred pounds, I presumed my next question might be foolhardy, but I took the risk. "How would you suggest I do that?" I asked hopefully. She stared at my journal as if she might find the answer there. It seemed that I had stumped her. "Go to bed at 7:15," she quipped.

Weight can be controlled only when there is a balance between calories consumed and energy expended. Exercise is an essential component of a weight maintenance program, but to start losing, calories have to be cut. And what if food answers more needs than nutrition?

Choosing substitute habits ahead of time will help ensure that the next stressful event doesn't bring on a binge. For meal planning and information on healthful eating, nutritionists or dieticians are great, but discovering a behavior that can replace eating and still give the desired effect may require different resources. Weight-loss groups such as Weight Watchers are helpful to many people because of both the support of the group and the shared ideas and solutions. Psychological counseling can help. Massage can be an effective tool for managing simple daily stress, as can a warm, soothing bath with a satisfying novel. Exercise of any type serves a dual purpose of both expending calories and maintaining a biochemical balance that reduces stress and symptoms of depression. For exercise, yoga, mediation, and other stress-reducing tools, most communities offer classes. The American Heart Association, the American Diabetes Association, and many other groups sponsor community walks, runs, or bicycle rides to raise money and awareness of their causes. Becoming involved in organizations and training for their outings is another great opportunity for not only improving health, but enjoying the satisfaction of contributing to the community.

If nothing seems to work and obesity is a genuine issue, a visit to a physician and insistence on help may be necessary. Underlying metabolic disorders should be investigated. There are prescription drugs available that have demonstrated moderate success, and for the person whose weight significantly impairs health, surgery may offer a lifesaving alternative.

Why do anything at all? In the larger picture, it will help ensure that the healthcare system remains viable, but that will hardly serve as an immediate motivator. Everyone has his own reason. Perhaps it is to reclaim an activity that used to be pleasurable, or to regain lost energy. Perhaps it is just to prove that it is still possible to get into those "skinny" pants that take up space in the back of a drawer, or to feel younger. Short of a fountain of youth, maintaining a healthy weight, eating healthy foods, and exercising regularly is the next best thing! Whatever the reason, taking action could prevent three hundred thousand premature deaths per year while relieving the pressure on an overburdened healthcare system.

Here are just a few Web sites to investigate for further information about weight control: www.obesity.org, www.weightwatchers.com, www.overeatersanonymous. org, and http://atkins.com.

Notes

1. Nanci Hellmich and Anita Manning, "Scales Tipping toward Diabetes: Twin Scourge of Weight and Disease Could 'Break the Bank' of Healthcare," *USA Today*, October 24, 2002. This article is no longer archived at the USA Today site, but it is available at www.defeatdiabetes.org/articles/obesity3021024.htm.

2. "The Surgeon General's Call to Action to Prevent and Decrease Overweight and Obesity," Virtual Office of the Surgeon General [online], www.surgeongeneral.gov/topics/obesity/calltoaction/fact_consequences.htm [January 2003].

3. Ibid.

4. Hellmich and Manning, "Scales Tipping toward Diabetes."

APPENDIX F
Information for Kids

*T*he *Magic Stethoscope*, a delightful book about nursing aimed at middle school–aged children, was written by a group of nurses enrolled in a writing class at George Mason University, under the direction of Jeanne Sorrell, PhD, RN. The book can be ordered by sending a check for $14 ($12 for book; $2 for postage), along with your mailing address to:

Jeanne M. Sorrell, PhD, RN
ATTENTION: Magic Stethoscope
College of Nursing and Health Science
MSN 3C4
George Mason University
4400 University Drive
Fairfax, VA 22030

Checks should be made out to "GMU—CNHS." Proceeds benefit a nursing scholarship fund at George Mason University. For information about the book, please contact Dr. Jeanne Sorrell at Jsorrell@gmu.edu or 703-993-1944.

The Virginia Partnership for Nursing has established an interactive Web site that offers information about nursing aimed at school grade levels K–3, 4–8, and 9–12.

For further information, visit their Web site at www.nurses-changelives.com.

Index